XENOTRANSPLANTATION

Edited by **Shuji Miyagawa**

Xenotransplantation
Edited by Shuji Miyagawa

Published by InTech
Janeza Trdine 9, 51000 Rijeka, Croatia

Publishing Process Manager Romana Vukelic

Technical Editor Teodora Smiljanic

Cover Designer InTech Design Team

Additional hard copies can be obtained from orders@intechopen.com

Xenotransplantation, Edited by Shuji Miyagawa
p. cm.
ISBN 978-953-307-997-4

For EU product safety concerns:
IN TECH d.o.o., Prolaz Marije Krucifikse Kozulić 3, 51000 Rijeka, Croatia,
info@intechopen.com or visit our website at intechopen.com.

Meet the editor

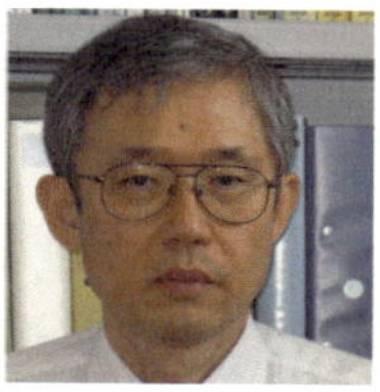

Dr Shuji Miyagawa is an Associate Professor of Surgery at the Osaka University Graduate School of Medicine, Japan. After graduating at Hokkaido University Medical School, he finished clinical training in the 1st Department of Surgery, Osaka University Medical School. He obtained his PhD in transplantation immunology from the same University in 1989. Dr Shuji Miyagawa worked at University of Texas Medical School in Houston as a Research Associate from 1988-1990. He became an Assistant Professor in 1995, and Associate Professor at the Osaka University in 1998. His works have been presented in numerous international meetings, especially International Xenotransplantation Association (IXA), and he sits on the editorial board of several international journals, such as Xenotransplantation.

Contents

Preface

Attempts of transplanting tissue from animals to humans have been made for hundreds of years. Several records are found from 17th Century. In the years to come, many clinical trials were done one after another. However, with the successful progress of allotransplantation using new immunosuppressive drugs, such as cyclosporine, the necessity of xenotransplantation has declined.

However, the current shortage of donor organs and the increasing need for them have led to a revival of interest in the area of xenotransplantation. Xenografting can be classified as either discordant or concordant, such as pig to human or monkey to human, respectively, based on the severity and pattern of the graft rejection. The pig represents an ideal animal for discordant xenografts due to a variety of reasons, including anatomical, physiological and ethical considerations. The exposure of pig cells, tissues and organs to human blood, however, results in a hyperacute rejection (HAR) which is mediated by naturally occurring high-titer antibodies, mainly a variety epitope Gal alpha(1,3)Gal and complements in humans.

After the transgenic technique became useful for pigs, transgenic (TG)-pigs with the complement regulatory proteins, such as decay accelerating factor (DAF: CD55), were produced in succession. Xenotransplantation study, for example the prevention of NK cell, an expression of HLA on pigs, also became popular all over the world.

However, once the problems of porcine endogenous retrovirus (PERVs) emerged, the boom of xenotransplantation study relatively declined. The pig genome contains at least 50 pro-viral copies of PERVs. The ability of PERV to infect human cells in vitro has generated a debate concerning the risks associated with xenotransplantation.

On the other hand, accompanied by the advent of animal cloning, the technique of nuclear transfer produced alpha1,3-galactosyltransferase-knockout (Gal-KO) pigs in many institutes, including Japan, at the beginning of 21st Century. In addition, the controversy about the risk of PERV has gradually minimized, because of the fact that there are no cases of PERV infections reported in humans. Furthermore, a large clinical wave of islet allotransplantation resumed the interest of xenotransplantation, especially porcine islet transplantation and some exceptions. Moreover, a new study of xenotransplantation for neurodegenerative diseases also started in Europe.

InTech started the book *Xenotransplantation* and invited me to be the editor, which was an honor to accept. The recent unpopularity of xenotransplantation studies and my relative influence in this field resulted with a number of chapters that are not as comprehensive to cover the full extent of xenotransplantation study at this time. However, the chapters gathered herein introduce extremely important topics.

Finally, the clinical trials were done in many countries so far, such as Sweden, China, Mexico, USA (Inventory of Human Xenotransplantation Practices: IXA and HUG in collaboration with WHO). In addition, a new clinical trial was approved by the government, and resumed the porcine islet transplantation research in New Zealand two years ago.

Dr. Shuji Miyagawa
Osaka University Graduate School of Medicine
Department of Surgery
Japan

Part 1

Basic

1

Anti-Gal and Anti-Non Gal Antibody Barriers in Xenotransplantation

Uri Galili
Department of Surgery, University of Massachusetts Medical School, Worcester
USA

1. Introduction

The many studies on the immune mechanisms contributing to xenograft rejection have identified two types of antibodies (Abs) that form barriers to transplantation of xenografts into humans: 1. Natural and induced anti-Gal Abs, and 2. Induced anti-non gal Abs. The formidable barrier of anti-Gal Abs seems to have been removed by the generation of α1,3galactosyltransferase (α1,3GT) knockout (KO) pigs. However, the second immune barrier of anti-non gal Abs may be even more formidable than that of anti-Gal Abs. The anti-non gal Ab barrier was not fully appreciated in the 1990's when much of the research was focused on overcoming the first barrier of anti-Gal mediated hyperacute rejection of pig xenografts. The anti-non gal Ab barrier still presents a challenge that requires the development of novel immunological treatments which prevent the production of these Abs. It is possible that without overcoming the anti-non gal Ab barrier it may be difficult to progress in clinical xenotransplantation beyond the use of short term bridge xenografts. Both the anti-Gal and anti-non gal barriers have been the focus of many studies in nonprimate mammal and in monkeys. This chapter does not intend to review the vast literature on anti-Gal and anti-non gal immune response in experimental animal models, but aims primarily to describe the information gained in studying anti-Gal and anti-non gal Ab response in humans. Although xenotransplantation is rarely performed in humans, I have had the opportunity of collaborating with several groups that introduced xenogeneic cells or tissues expressing α-gal epitopes into humans and study anti-Gal and anti-non gal Ab response in the sera of such patients. I believe that the information gained in these studies may contribute to the understanding of the immune response to α-gal epitopes and to xenoantigens that induce the anti-non gal Ab response in humans.

2. The anti-Gal Ab and the α-gal epitope

Anti-Gal is the most abundant Ab in humans, comprising ~1% of circulating immunoglobulins (Galili et al., 1984). This Ab is present in the serum as IgG, IgM and IgA isotypes and in various body secretions as IgG and IgA (Galili et al., 1984; Hamadeh et al., 1995; Yu et al., 1999). In recent studies, anti-Gal was found in some individuals also as an IgE Ab that can mediate a systemic allergic reaction following the infusion of the monoclonal Ab cetuximab which carries α-gal epitopes on its Fab (Chung et al. 2008). The isotype switch into anti-Gal IgE was reported to be associated with biting of the tick *Amblyomma americanum* which transmits lime disease (Commins et al., 2011). Although anti-Gal is present in large amounts in humans it interacts with a very high specificity with a carbohydrate antigen (Ag) called the α-gal epitope (Galα1-3Galβ1-4GlcNAc-R) on glycolipids and glycoproteins (Galili et al., 1985; 1987a). Anti-Gal is produced in humans throughout life as a result of continuous antigenic stimulation by gastrointestinal bacteria with cell wall carbohydrate Ags that have a structure similar to the α-gal epitope (Galili et al. 1988a). Anti-blood group A and B Abs are also produced as a result of antigenic stimulation by the gastrointestinal flora (Springer & Horton, 1969). However, anti-Gal differs from these blood group Abs in that it is produced in all humans who are not severely immunocompromized. In individuals with blood type A and O, >80% of anti-blood group B activity is in fact by anti-Gal Abs that are capable of binding to α-gal epitopes despite of the branching fucose, as in blood group B Ag (i.e. Galα1-3(Fucα1-2)Galβ1-4GlcNAc-R) (Galili et al., 1987a; McMorrow et al., 1997). However, in blood group B and AB individuals, anti-Gal exclusively interacts with the α-gal epitope and not with other carbohydrate structures.

In contrast to protein Ags, carbohydrate Ags (with the exception of sialic acid) have no electrostatic charges. Therefore the affinity of anti-Gal to the α-gal epitope is much lower than that of anti-protein Abs. Affinity analysis performed by equilibrium dialysis using free α-gal epitope as the radiolabeled trisaccharide [^{3}H]Galα1-3Galβ1-4GlcNAc have indicated that the affinity is highly variable in different individuals and it ranges between $2x10^5$ to $6x10^6M^{-1}$ (Galili & Matta, 1996). However, since anti-Gal is produced in very large amounts, it is very effective in inducing destruction of pig cells and tissues expressing α-gal epitopes on their surface (Galili, 1993; Good et al., 1992; Sandrin et al., 1993; Collins et al., 1994).

The proportion of B cells capable of producing anti-Gal is ~1% of circulating B cells, whereas the proportion of B cells capable of producing anti-blood group A or B Abs is 4-5 fold lower (Galili et al., 1992). This could be determined by immortalization of human blood B cells by Epstein Barr virus and the growth of such cells as individual clones. One in 100 B cells produces anti-Gal *in vitro* whereas only one in 400-500 B cell clones produces anti-blood group A or B Abs (Galili et al., 1993). Most of B cells capable of producing the anti-Gal Ab (designated anti-Gal B cells) are quiescent and only those along the gastrointestinal tract continuously produce this natural Ab. Analysis of the immunoglobulin genes in anti-Gal B cells indicated that this is a polyclonal population, however, the immunoglobulin heavy chain genes in most clones, cluster in the VH3 family (Wang et al., 1995).

3. Distribution of the α-gal epitope and anti-Gal Ab in mammals

The α-gal epitope is unique to mammals, where it is found as $1x10^6$-$30x10^6$ epitopes/cell and is completely absent in fish, amphibians, reptiles, or birds (Galili et al., 1987b, 1988b). Among mammals, α-gal epitopes are present on cells of marsupials such as kangaroo and opossum and on cells of non-primate placental mammals like mouse, rat, rabbit, bat, pig, cow, horse, cat, dog, and dolphin (Galili et al. 1987b, 1988b). The α-gal epitope is also found in similar abundance on cells of prosimians (e.g., lemurs), and New World monkeys (i.e., monkeys of South America), but not on cells of Old World monkeys (monkeys of Asia and Africa), apes (e.g., chimpanzee, gorilla and orangutan), and humans (Galili et al., 1987b, 1988b). In contrast, humans, apes and Old World monkeys are not immunotolerant to the α-gal epitope and they all produce large amounts of the natural anti-Gal Ab against it (Galili et al., 1987b).

The unique distribution of α-gal epitopes and the anti-Gal Ab in mammals is the result of the differential activity of the glycosylation enzyme α1,3galactosyltransferase (α1,3GT) which is active in the trans-Golgi compartment where it transfers galactose from the sugar donor UDP-Gal to N-acetyllactosamine (Galβ1-4GlcNAc-R) on carbohydrate chains of glycoproteins and glycolipids to synthesize the α-gal epitope. The α1,3GT gene (also referred to as *Ggta1*) is expressed in mammalian cells but is inactive in humans, apes and Old World monkeys (Galili et al. 1988b; Thall et al. 1991). This inactivation is primarily the result of various deletions in the *Ggta1* gene causing frame shift mutations in the open reading frame and the generation of pre-mature stop codons (Larsen et al., 1990; Joziasse et al., 1992; Galili & Swanson, 1992; Koike et al., 2002). Studies evaluating the expression of this pseudo-gene in humans by PCR have demonstrated its low transcription (Koike et al., 2002), however, since the protein molecule is truncated, it is devoid of catalytic activity. Truncation studies in the New World monkey α1,3GT have indicated that deletion of as few as three amino acids at the C-terminus is sufficient to result in complete lose of catalytic activity (Henion et al., 1994). Comparison of the sequence of this pseudogene in humans and in other primates led us to suggest that the α1,3GT gene was inactivated in ancestral Old World primates, after apes and monkeys diverged from each other, 20-25 million years ago (Galili & Swanson, 1992; Galili & Andrews, 1995).

4. The rejection of xenografts by the anti-Gal Ab

Several seminal studies demonstrated *in vitro* the destruction of cells by complement mediated cytolysis (Good et al., 1992, Sandrin et al., 1993) or by Ab dependent cell mediated cytotoxicity (ADCC) (Galili, 1993; Watier et al., 1996) due to interaction of human anti-Gal Ab with α-gal epitopes on pig cells or on monkey cells transfected with α1,3GT gene and thus expressing the α-gal epitopes on their cell membrane. In *in vivo* studies, transplantation of pig or New World monkey xenografts into Old World monkeys was found to result in *in situ* binding of anti-Gal to α-gal epitopes on endothelial cells of grafts, complement mediated lysis of these cells due to this Ag/Ab interaction, the ensuing collapse of the vascular bed and hyper acute rejection of the xenograft (Collins et al., 1994). Subsequent studies demonstrated the direct association between *in vivo* neutralization of anti-Gal by α-gal oligosaccharides and delay in hyperacute rejection (Simon et al., 1998), and the association between removal of anti-Gal by adsorption on affinity columns and delay in xenograft rejection (Kozlowski et al., 1998; Xu et al., 1998). These studies directly proved that the anti-Gal Ab is the Ab mediating hyperacute rejection of xenogafts *in vivo*.

5. Stimulation of the immune system to produce anti-Gal Ab in xenograft recipients

Anti-Gal is present in very high amounts in all individuals who are not severely immunocompromized. Nevertheless, the human immune system is capable of producing this Ab in much higher titers due to the activation of many of the quiescent anti-Gal B cells throughout the body. As indicated above, ~1% of B cells in the blood have the capacity of producing the anti-Gal Ab, but are in a quiescent state (Galili et al., 1993). However, in individuals who are transplanted with xenografts that present α-gal epitopes, these quiescent B cells are readily activated to produce the anti-Gal Ab. The activated anti-Gal B cells further undergo isotype switch as well as affinity maturation, ultimately resulting in an increase of ~100 fold in the titer of this Ab.

Anti-Gal Ab response to α-gal epitopes on xenogeneic cells could be monitored in an ovarian carcinoma patient who received an experimental gene therapy treatment for destruction of tumor cells by ganciclovir (Galili et al., 2001). The patient received 3 intraperitoneal infusions in 7 weeks intervals, each of $6x10^9$ mouse fibroblasts that released a replication defective retro-virus containing the thymidine kinase gene. Tumor cells infected *in situ* by the virus are killed by subsequent administration of ganciclovir (Link et al., 1996). Since the infused mouse fibroblasts present multiple α-gal epitopes (Galili et al., 1988b), this treatment is immunologically similar to the transplantation of xenograft cells expressing α-gal epitopes in humans. Anti-Gal activity in the serum of the patient was studied by ELISA with synthetic α-gal epitopes linked to bovine serum albumin (α-gal BSA) as solid phase Ag. Within one week post infusion of mouse fibroblasts, the titer of anti-Gal IgG Ab increased by ~10 fold, and two weeks post post infusion by ~100 fold (Galili et al., 2001) (Fig. 1). The Ab activity remained at that high level after the second and third infusions. This extensive anti-Gal Ab response was the result of activation of the many anti-Gal B cell clones that engage α-gal epitopes on the glycoproteins released from the infused mouse fibroblasts. Studies measuring the concentration of anti-Gal in the serum (by isolation on an α-gal column) and its affinity (by dialysis of radiolabled free α-gal epitope in the form of trisaccharide [Galili & Matta, 1996]) indicated that the 10 fold increase in anti-Gal titer within the first week post transplantation was the result of an increase in the concentration of anti-Gal Ab in the serum (i.e. increased production of the Ab), whereas the additional 10 fold increase within the second week was associated with a corresponding increase in the affinity of this Ab (Galili et al., 2001). These findings strongly suggest that the increase in the titer of anti-Gal Ab observed after one week is the result of activation of quiescent anti-Gal B cells by α-gal epitopes on glycoproteins released from the xenograft cells, thereby increasing the concentration of this Ab in the serum. The subsequent increase in affinity of the Ab observed at the end of the second week is probably a result of affinity maturation by the process of somatic mutations within anti-Gal B cell clones. This process occurs after the initial activation of the quiescent anti-Gal B cells.

The increase in anti-Gal Ab response was mostly (~90%) of the IgG2 subclass and the remaining was of the IgG3 subclass. No significant increase was observed in the activity of anti-Gal IgG1, IgG4, IgM or IgA (Galili et al., 2001). This suggests that the isotype switch of anti-Gal B cells stimulated by α-gal presenting xenoglycoproteins (α-gal glycoproteins) is quite rapid from IgM to IgG2 and IgG3. It should be stressed, however, that anti-Gal IgM is naturally present in large amounts in human serum (Hamadeh et al., 1995; Yu et al., 1999) and anti-Gal IgA and IgG are present in various secretion such as saliva, milk, colostrum and bile (Hamadeh et al., 1995).

Activation of anti-Gal B cells and production of the anti-Gal Ab by plasma cells seems to occur as long as there are glycoproteins with α-gal epitopes in the body. The decrease in anti-Gal titer observed 4 and 7 weeks after the first infusion of mouse fibroblasts (Fig. 1) suggests that after the anti-Gal mediated destruction of these cells and the elimination of α-gal glycoproteins, anti-Gal B cells cease to be activated and to differentiate into plasma cells secreting the Ab. Since the period of Ab secretion by plasma cells is limited, activity of anti-Gal Ab decreases in the serum within a short period after the elimination of glycoproteins with α-gal epitopes. It is of interest to note that anti-Gal production after the second and third infusions of mouse fibroblasts was not higher than that observed after the first infusion (Fig. 1). It is probable that high affinity anti-Gal IgG molecules produced in large amounts, effectively mask α-gal epitopes on glycoproteins released from the infused cells. Such masking limits the extent of further B cell activation and keeps that activation at a level of Ab production similar to that observed 2 weeks after the first infusion.

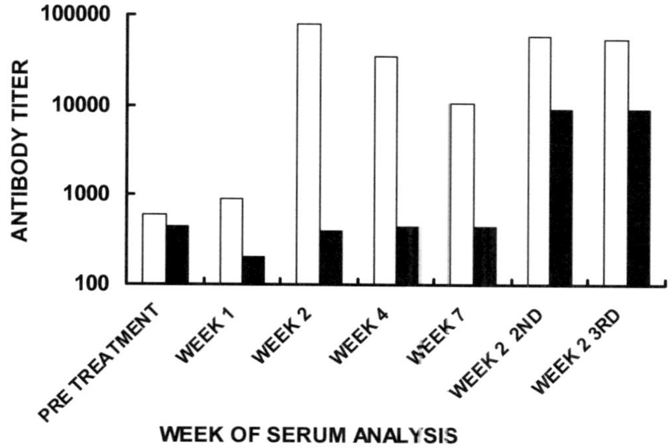

Fig. 1. Production of anti-Gal (open columns) and anti-non gal IgG Abs (closed columns) in an ovarian carcinoma recipient of $6x10^9$ mouse fibroblasts. The patient received 3 intraperitoneal infusions of the fibroblasts in 7 week intervals. Ab titers were determined prior to treatment, 1, 2, 4 and 7 weeks post treatment, 2 weeks after the second (2nd) and third (3rd) treatments. The titers are presented as reciprocals of serum dilution yielding half the maximum binding in ELISA. The solid phase Ags used for the study were synthetic α-gal epitopes linked to BSA (α-gal BSA) for anti-Gal Ab analysis and the mouse fibroblast cell line used in the treatment for anti-non gal Ab analysis. Sera were depleted of anti-Gal Ab prior to performing the assay for anti-non gal Abs (modified from Galili et al., 2001).

A similar extensive increase in anti-Gal titer was observed in patients with impaired liver function, who were treated by temporary extracorporeal perfusion of their blood through a pig liver (Cotterell et al., 1995; Yu et al. 1999). The increase in anti-Gal titer in these patients implies that the release of xenoglycoproteins from the pig liver, perfused for several hours, was sufficient to induce the activation of the many quiescent anti-Gal B cells for production of the anti-Gal Ab. Interestingly, a similar rapid and extensive increase in anti-Gal IgG activity was observed in cynomolgus monkeys (an Old World monkey) implanted with pig meniscus cartilage which contains an abundance of α-gal epitopes (Galili et al., 1997). This suggests that non-human primates capable of producing anti-Gal Ab also have multiple quiescent anti-Gal B cells as those in humans.

6. Anti-Gal Ab production in immunosuppressed xenograft recipients

The extensive activation of anti-Gal B cells by α-gal epitopes on xenografts is very difficult to suppress. This can be inferred from the studies on anti-Gal response in diabetic patients who were transplanted by Groth and colleagues with an allogeneic kidney together with pig fetal islet cell clusters (Groth et al., 1994; Galili et al., 1995). These studies were the first to demonstrate the induced anti-Gal Ab response in xenograft recipients. Pig islet cell clusters were generated by culturing of fetal pig pancreatic tissues (Korsgren et al. 1988). The fetal islet cells proliferate *in vitro* and form clusters of islet cells which were transplanted at a volume corresponding to 2-6 ml packed cells (Groth et al., 1994). The islet cell clusters were implanted under the transplanted kidney capsule or infused into the portal vein in the liver. Recipients of the kidney allograft and the islet cell xenografts displayed an increase of 20-80 folds in anti-Gal titer within the period of 25-50 days post transplantation (Galili et al., 1995). As with the ovarian carcinoma patient infused intraperitoneal with the mouse fibroblasts (Galili et al., 2001), the increase in anti-Gal activity was mostly in the IgG isotype and to a much lesser extent of IgM and IgA isotypes. However, unlike the ovarian carcinoma patient, the transplanted diabetic patients were heavily immunosuppressed, to the extent that the immune system did not reject the kidney allograft (Groth et al., 1994). The increased production of anti-Gal Ab in these immunosuppressed patients suggests that currently used immunosuppressive protocols, which are effective enough to prevent allograft rejection, fail in preventing much of the activation of anti-Gal B cells by α-gal glycoproteins released from the xenograft.

Studies in α1,3galactosyltransferase knockout mice that are capable of producing anti-Gal Ab have indicated that stimulation of anti-Gal B cells by α-gal epitopes on xenografts to produce the anti-Gal Ab requires T cell help. However, the α-gal epitope by itself (like other carbohydrate chains of the complex type) can not activate helper T cells (Tanemura et al., 2000). T cell help for anti-Gal B cells is provides by helper T cells activated by the multiple xenogeneic peptides processed and presented by antigen presenting cells (Tanemura et al., 2000; Galili 2004). Interestingly, in the absence of T cell help, interaction between α-gal epitopes and B cell receptors on anti-Gal B cells results in induction of immune tolerance to α-gal epitopes and prevention of anti-Gal Ab production in the tolerized recipients (Mohiuddin et al., 2003; Ogawa et al., 2003). A similar tolerance induction was achieved by bone marrow chimerism with α-gal epitope presenting syngeneic bone marrow cells (Bracy et al., 1998).

7. Elimination of the anti-Gal Ab barrier by the use of α1,3galactosyltransferase knockout pigs

As indicated above, the natural anti-Gal Ab and the elicited anti-Gal Ab are of no clinic significance in xenograft recipients, if the xenograft is obtained from α1,3galactosyltransferase knockout pigs. These pigs have been generated by targeted disruption (knockout) of the α1,3galactosyltransferase gene (Phelps et al., 2003; Kobler-Simond et al., 2004; Yamada et al., 2005; Takahagi et al., 2005; McGregor et al., 2011). These pigs lack α-gal epitopes and their organs do not induce an anti-Gal response when transplanted into primates (Chen et al., 2005; Ezzelarab et al., 2006; Hisashi et al., 2008; Yeh et al., 2010). Thus, in contrast to rapid (hyperacute) rejection of wild type (WT) pig organs in monkeys (observed within <1h to several hours), pig organs from α1,3galactosyltransferase knockout pigs (α1,3GT KO pigs) survive in monkeys for weeks to several months prior to rejection (Yamada et al., 2005; Chen et al., 2005; Kuwaki et al., 2005; Tseng et al., 2005; Hisashi et al., 2008). In the absence of anti-Gal response the next immune obstacle in xenotransplantation became apparent- the production of anti-non gal Abs against xenoantigens of the graft which are not α-gal epitopes. Most of these xenoantigens are multiple pig proteins that are immunogenic in humans.

8. Most of the proteins within pig xenografts are expected to be immunogenic in humans

The amino acid sequence of most homologous (orthologous) proteins varies in different mammals. There are only few highly conserved proteins, such as histones and collagen in which amino acid sequence changes have been minimal because of functional constraints. However, most genes accumulate random mutations (referred to as the evolutionary molecular clock [Wilson & Sarich, 1969]) which result in variations in amino acid sequence. Since humans and pigs (as well as other nonprimate mammals) have been evolving independently along separate lineages for an evolutionary period estimated to be ~75 million years (Pilbeam 1984), each has accumulated multiple lineage and species specific mutations. The proportion of such mutations varies in different regions of a given protein, based on functional constraints, e.g. in a membrane bound receptor there are more mutations in the tether region than the ligand binding region. Regardless of their location, mutations form immunogenic amino acid sequences in pig proteins, since they are absent in humans. The immune system can react against very small changes in various Ags. This can be inferred from the immune response to blood group Ags where the presence of one small N-acetyl group (CH_3CONH) in blood group A and its absence in blood group B is sufficient for inducing production of anti-A Abs in blood group B individuals. Because most pig proteins contain some amino acid sequences that are different from those in homologous proteins in humans, it is likely that most pig proteins are immunogenic in humans and can induce an Ab response in xenograft recipients. Therefore, humans transplanted with pig cells or organs may produce hundreds and possibly thousands of Ab specificities against pig xenogeneic peptides. These Abs have been referred to as anti-non gal Abs (Galili et al., 2001). Since there are very large numbers of undefined xenoantigens that elicit anti-non gal Ab response, pig tissues or cells may serve as antigenic preparations for analysis of such Abs. For such analysis, anti-Gal Abs have to be removed from the tested human sera prior to the assay. This anti-Gal depletion is feasible by adsorption of anti-Gal Ab on rabbit RBC or on glutaraldehyde rabbit RBC (Galili et al., 2001; Stone et al., 2007) since these RBC present the highest number of α-gal epitopes among mammalian RBC (Ogawa & Galili, 2006). As described below, studies on anti-non gal Abs in xenograft recipients have indicated that their production is very different from that of elicited anti-Gal Abs.

9. Anti-non gal Abs in a recipient of mouse fibroblasts

The studies on the Ab response in the ovarian carcinoma patient receiving intraperitoneal infusion of mouse fibroblasts led to the first report on production of anti-non gal Abs in humans that are recipients of a xenograft (Galili et al. 2001). Although, in this patient the anti-non gal Ab response was against mouse proteins, the results of this analysis are also applicable to the understanding of anti-non gal immune response to pig proteins. This is since the evolutionary distance between humans and rodents does not differ significantly from the distance between humans and pigs (i.e. ~75 million years of evolution in separate lineages since the "great mammalian radiation") [Pilbeam 1984]. Anti-non gal Ab activity in that patient could be determined by ELISA with the mouse fibroblast cell line used in the treatment, as a solid phase Ag. These fibroblasts strongly adhere to ELISA wells following the overnight drying of the cell suspension in the wells. Serum samples from various time points post intraperitoneal infusion were the same as those used for anti-Gal analysis (Fig. 1), however, the sera were depleted of anti-Gal Abs by adsorption on rabbit RBC (50%) on ice (Galili et al., 2001).

Although anti-Gal IgG Ab activity increased by ~14 days post administration of the mouse fibroblasts, no induced anti-non gal Ab production was detected at that time point (Fig. 1). These Abs were not detected even 7 weeks after the first infusion. However, within 2 weeks after the second infusion, a robust anti-non gal Ab response was observed in the serum of the patient (Fig. 1). Western blot analysis indicated that the Abs produced bound to multiple proteins in the mouse fibroblasts, confirming the multiclonality of the B cell response (Galili et al. 2001). It is probable that there are also many T cell clones that are activated by xenogeneic peptides processed and presented by the antigen presenting cells of the treated patient. Nevertheless, the lack of detectable induced anti-non gal Ab response after the first fibroblast infusion strongly supports the assumption that the initial number of anti-non gal B cells in each of the multiple B cell clones reacting against xenoantigens is very low. By the time B cells in these multiple clones proliferate to the extent required for producing detectable levels of anti-non gal Abs, the stimulatory fibroblasts have disappeared due to anti-Gal Ab mediated destruction. Thus, production of anti-non gal Abs is detectable only after the second infusion of mouse fibroblasts which provides an antigenic boost for the activation of anti-non gal memory B cells. As shown below, anti-non gal Abs appear at earlier time point in recipients of pig tissue (tendon) because of the continuous antigenic stimulation by the pig xenoantigens. The subclass distribution of the induced anti-non gal Abs was found to be IgG1>IgG2>IgG3>IgG4 (Galili et al. 2001).

It is of interest to note that the titer of anti-non gal Abs measured after the third infusion (performed 7 weeks post second infusion) did not differ from that after the second infusion (Fig. 1). These observations strongly suggests that, as with anti-Gal Ab response, anti-non gal Ab response is subjected to a self limiting dynamic regulatory mechanism. This self limiting production of anti-non gal Abs may be mediated by such Ab molecules that bind to the immunogenic peptide epitopes and mask them, thereby preventing additional stimulation of the corresponding B cells.

10. Anti-non gal Ab response in recipients of pig ligament

A phase I clinical trial on replacement of torn anterior cruciate ligament (ACL) with pig patellar tendon provided a unique opportunity for monitoring anti-non gal Ab response in the absence of immunosuppression in humans, for a period of 2 years (Stone et al. 2007). The implanted ligaments and the two attached bone blocks were treated with recombinant α-galactosidase in order to eliminate α-gal epitopes. This enzymatic treatment was performed in order to attenuate the immune response to the implant by preventing the induction of anti-Gal Ab response which can be detrimental to the implant. In addition, the ligaments underwent mild cross-linking by incubation for 12 hours with 0.1% glutaraldehyde. It was assumed that in the absence of anti-Gal response, destruction of the pig ligament mediated by anti-non gal Abs will be slowed due to the cross-linking. The slowed destruction of the cross-linked ligament will enable concomitant regeneration of the ligament tissue (ligamentization) by infiltrating fibroblasts which align with the pig collagen fiber scaffold and produce new collagen fibers. It was further assumed that the similarity in the rates of pig ligament destruction and ligamentization by human fibroblasts will maintain the biomechanical characteristics of the implanted ligament while it is gradually replaced by the human tissue. Five patients receiving such implants 9-10 years ago continue to display normal joint activity.

Anti-non gal Ab response was studied in implanted patients by ELISA with pig ligament homogenate as solid phase Ag, using sera that were depleted of anti-Gal Ab. Induction of anti-non gal Ab production was determined by comparison of the post-implantation Ab activity at various serum dilutions with that in the pre-implantation base-line activity. The induced anti-non gal Ab response peaked 2 - 6 months post implantation (Fig. 2) (Stone et al. 2007). This Ab response was detectable also after 1 year, but it returned to the pre-implantation level after 2 years. These observations suggest that as long as the pig tissue is present within the recipient, the immune system is stimulated to produce anti-non gal Abs. However, due to the gradual replacement with human ligament tissue, the amount of pig ligament tissue is decreasing, so that by 12 months anti-non gal Ab response is lower than in the peak of 2-6 months. By 24 months, the pig ligament seems to be completely replaced by human ligament tissue therefore there is no antigenic stimulation for the production of anti-non gal Abs.

Anti-non gal IgG Ab activity in the pig ligament recipients increased on average by 5-10 folds in comparison with pre-implantation serum in each of the patients (Stone et al., 2007). This increase is much lower than the ~100 fold increase in anti-Gal Ab activity observed in the patient receiving intraperitoneal infusion of mouse fibroblasts. The difference is likely to be due to the much higher number of quiescent anti-Gal B cells (~1% of B cells [Galili et al., 1993]) which are rapidly activated by α-gal epitopes on xenoglycoproteins. The ultimate number of anti-non gal B cells at the peak of the immune response is likely to be much lower in each of the individual clones, thus, the overall immune response is significantly lower than that of the anti-Gal response.

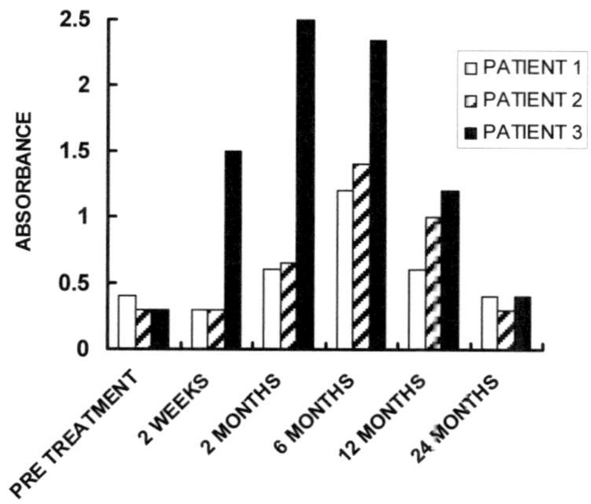

Fig. 2. Anti-non gal Ab (IgG) activity in the sera of 3 patients implanted with pig patellar tendon for replacement of torn ACL. The pig tendons were treated with α-galactosidase for destruction of α-gal epitopes and cross-linked mildly with glutaraldehyde prior to implantation. Ab activity was determined by ELISA with pig ligament homogenate as solid phase Ag. Sera were depleted of anti-Gal Ab prior to analysis. Ab binding was determined at serum dilution of 1:640 and presented as O.D. (optical density units) at the various time points (modified from Stone et al., 2007).

The specificity of the anti-non gal Abs could be studied by Western blots. Pre-implantation sera depleted of anti-Gal Abs displayed no Ab binding to pig ligament proteins or to pig kidney proteins. However, sera obtained 6 months post implantation contained anti-non gal Abs that bound to multiple pig ligament proteins. This large number of Ab specificities was indicated by the immunostaining of the blot as a smear rather than as individual bands (Stone et al., 2007). Many of stained proteins were also found in pig kidney preparations, implying that some of the proteins inducing anti-non gal Ab response are not specific to the ligament and are present in other tissues, as well. Blots of human ligament proteins were also studied for binding of anti-non gal IgG Abs. Despite the extensive binding of Abs to pig ligament proteins, no binding was observed with human ligament proteins. This strongly suggests that exposure of the human immune system to pig proteins and the extensive production of Abs against such proteins does not result in breakdown of immune tolerance to self Ags and no auto-Abs are generated.

It is not clear as yet whether the anti-non gal Ab response also includes Abs to carbohydrate Ags other than the α-gal epitope. A number of studies demonstrated the production of natural Abs to N-glycolylneuraminic acid in humans and the presence this epitope on pig cells (Zhu & Hurst, 2002; Miwa et al., 2004; Taylor et al., 2010). However, analysis of sera from monkeys sensitized to α1,3GT KO pig tissue demonstrated no significant elevation in the activity of such Abs (Yeh et al., 2010).

11. Anti-non gal Ab response in immunosuppressed recipients

The study of sera in diabetic recipients of pig fetal islet cell clusters enabled the assessment of anti-non gal Ab production in recipients of pig fetal islet cell xenograft and of a kidney allograft. These recipients were immunosuppressed to the extent that they did not reject the allograft (Groth et al., 1994). As indicated above, the immunosuppressive treatment in these patients did not prevent the induced anti-Gal immune response against α-gal epitopes on xenoglycoproteins. In order to estimate the proportion of anti-Gal and anti-non gal Abs of the total Ab binding to pig cells, binding of IgG Abs to pig PK15 kidney cells was measured in serum of transplanted patients and compared to the binding of Abs after anti-Gal depletion by binding of the Ab to α-gal epitopes linked to silica beads. Ab binding to pig cells in serum depleted of anti-Gal was 6-25% of the total IgG binding (Galili et al., 1995). These findings suggest that anti-Gal response comprised the majority of the human immune response to pig xenograft. Nevertheless, a significant proportion of the Abs was anti-non gal Abs produced despite immunosuppression effective enough to prevent the rejection of the kidney allograft.

Anti-non gal Ab production in the immunosuppressed recipients of kidney allograft and pig islet cell xenografts raises the question of whether these Abs are potent enough to mediate rejection of the xenograft. There is no direct information to address this question. Studies of xenotransplantation under immunosuppression of wild type pig heart and kidney into monkeys demonstrated anti-non gal Ab production, even if the xenograft was rejected within few days (Buhler et al., 2003; Lam et al., 2004; Chen et al., 2005; Ezzelarab et al., 2006). Transplantation of α1,3GT KO pig heart or kidney in monkeys subjected to a variety of immunosuppressive protocols resulted in survival of the xenografts for much longer periods (from several days up to 3 months [even up to 6 months in one recipient of heart xenograft]) than survival of xenografts from wild type pigs presenting multiple α-gal epitopes (Kuwaki et al., 2005; Chen et al., 2005; Tseng et al., 2005; Chen et al., 2006; Ezzelarab et al., 2006; Hisashi et al., 2008). Ultimately, all xenografts were rejected and the recipient monkeys were found to produce anti-non gal Abs which could be detected *in vitro* as Abs binding to α1,3GT KO pig cells. Although not directly proven, it is probable that these anti-non gal Abs contribute significantly to the observed rejection of α1,3GT KO pig xenografts.

12. Challenges in preventing anti-non gal Ab response in xenograft recipients

The prevention of anti-non gal Ab response in a xenograft recipient is a formidable challenge. As discussed above, this Ab response is the result of activation of multiple B cell clones against a very large number of immunogenic peptides on many pig proteins. It is probable that the multiple immunogenic peptides processed and presented by antigen presenting cells activate a very large number of helper T cell clones that facilitate anti-non gal Ab response. The studies mentioned above, which have demonstrated anti-non gal Ab response in immunosuppressed pig xenograft recipient monkeys imply that the immunosuppression protocols presently used for preventing allograft rejection do not completely prevent anti-non gal Ab response. Thus, a major challenge in xenotransplantation is the development of immunosuppressive drugs and protocols that prevent anti-non gal immune response but do not completely eliminate the ability of the immune system to protect against microbial pathogens. It is not clear at present whether such a selective immune suppression against multiple xenoantigens but not against microbial Ags is feasible. An alternative approach for preventing anti-non gal Ab response may be the induction of immune tolerance to the multiple pig xenoantigens. One method studied for inducing such a tolerance in kidney xenograft recipients has been the thymo-kidney xenograft of α1,3GT KO pigs (Yamada et al., 2005). Pig thymus tissue is placed under the pig kidney capsule several weeks prior to transplantation in order to achieve vascularization of this tissue. The thymus component of the xenograft is expected to tolerize the recipient against pig xenoantigens (Yamada et al., 2005). Pig thymo-kidney xenografts that were transplanted into monkey recipients survived for almost 3 months, a much longer period than the survival period of kidney xenografts lacking the thymus component (Yamada et al., 2005; Griesemer et al., 2009).

It may be possible that xenograft recipients will ultimately have to be tolerized to pig xenoantigens by manipulating their immune system prior to the xenotransplantation procedure. One theoretical possibility may be the effective pre-transplantation elimination of B cells of the patients. Newly emerging B cell clones with anti-pig Ag specificity that develop in the presence of the xenograft Ags (i.e. post transplantation) may be deleted from the repertoire at the differentiation stage of immature B cells in which B cells engaging Ags are eliminated or undergo receptor editing (Sandel & Monroe 1999; Nemazee et al., 2000). It is not known at present whether elimination of these B cells will suffice for preventing rejection, or is T cell elimination required as well. An additional tolerance induction method that is being explored is the administration of pig bone marrow cells in order to induce bone marrow chimerism which may prevent an immune response to pig xenoantigens. α1,3GT KO pig bone marrow cells were reported to survive in two out of four monkeys for at least 4 weeks (Griesemer et al., 2010). It is not known as yet whether such chimerism can be maintained for much longer periods and if it can prevent anti-non gal Ab response. In addition, it is not clear whether such chimerism can tolerize against xenoantigens that are not present on bone marrow cells (e.g. Ags specific to the pig xenograft organ). All these considerations imply that although the anti-Gal barrier has been effectively overcome, much research is still required for developing methods to overcome the anti-non gal immune response against the wide range of pig xenoantigens that are immunogenic in humans.

13. Concluding remarks

Two types of Abs form immune barriers in xenotransplantation: anti-Gal and anti-non gal Abs. The anti-Gal Ab is naturally present in humans in large amounts. The titer of anti-Gal Ab further increases in xenograft recipients by 30-100 fold because of the rapid activation of quiescent anti-Gal B cells which comprise ~1% of circulating B cells in humans. Production of anti-non gal Abs in xenograft recipients is the result of the immune response against the multiple pig proteins that are immunogenic in humans because of mutations in orthologous pig proteins. Anti-non gal Abs are produced by a large number of B cell clones with Ab specificity to the many pig peptide sequences that are not present in humans. Both anti-Gal and anti-non gal Abs are produced in humans despite immune suppression that is effective enough in preventing allograft rejection. Anti-Gal and anti-non gal Abs are continuously produced as long as the corresponding Ags are present in the treated patient. The generation of α1,3galactosyltransferase knockout pigs enabled the elimination of anti-Gal barrier in xenotransplantation since these pigs lack α-gal epitopes. However, overcoming the anti-non gal Ab barrier requires the development of novel methods that selectively prevent the induced production of these Abs while maintaining protective immune response against various pathogens.

14. References

Bracy JL, Sachs DH & Iacomini J. (1998) Inhibition of xenoreactive natural antibody production by retroviral gene therapy. *Science* 281:845-47.

Buhler L, Xu Y, Li W, Zhu A & Cooper DK. (2003) An investigation of the specificity of induced anti-pig antibodies in baboons. *Xenotransplantation*. 10:88-93.

Chen G, Qian H, Starzl T, Sun H, Garcia B, Wang X, Wise Y, Liu Y, Xiang Y, Copeman L, Liu W, Jevnikar A, Wall W, Cooper DK, Murase N, Dai Y, Wang W, Xiong Y, White DJ & Zhong R. (2005) Acute rejection is associated with antibodies to non-Gal antigens in baboons using Gal-knockout pig kidneys. *Nat Med.* 11:1295-8.

Chen G, Sun H, Yang H, Kubelik D, Garcia B, Luo Y, Xiang Y, Qian A, Copeman L, Liu W, Cardella CJ, Wang W, Xiong Y, Wall W, White DJ & Zhong R. (2006) The role of anti-non-Gal antibodies in the development of acute humoral xenograft rejection of hDAF transgenic porcine kidneys in baboons receiving anti-Gal antibody neutralization therapy. *Transplantation*. 81:273-83.

Chung CH, Mirakhur B, Chan E, Le QT, Berlin J, Morse M, Murphy BA, Satinover SM, Hosen J, Mauro D, Slebos RJ, Zhou Q, Gold D, Hatley T, Hicklin DJ & Platts-Mills TA. (2008) Cetuximab-induced anaphylaxis and IgE specific for galactose-α-1,3-galactose. *N Engl J Med.* 358::1109-17.

Collins BH, Cotterell AH, McCurry KR, Alvarado CG, Magee JC, Parker W &Platt JL. (1995) Cardiac xenografts between primate species provide evidence for the importance of the α-galactosyl determinant in hyperacute rejection. *J. Immunol.* 154: 5500-10.

Commins SP, James HR, Kelly LA, Pochan SL, Workman LJ, Perzanowski MS, Kocan KM, Fahy JV, Nganga LW, Ronmark E, Cooper PJ & Platts-Mills TA. (2011) The relevance of tick bites to the production of IgE antibodies to the mammalian oligosaccharide galactose-α-1,3-galactose. *J Allergy Clin Immunol*. 127:1286-93.

Cotterell AH, Collins BH, Parker W, Harland RC & Platt JL. (1995) The humoral immune response in humans following cross-perfusion of porcine organs. *Transplantation* 60:861-68.

Ezzelarab M, Hara H, Busch J, Rood PP, Zhu X, Ibrahim Z, Ball S, Ayares D, Awwad M & Cooper DK. (2006) Antibodies directed to pig non-Gal antigens in naïve and sensitized baboons. *Xenotransplantation*. 13:400-7.

Galili U & Andrews P. (1995) Suppression of α-galactosyl epitopes synthesis and production of the natural anti-Gal antibody: A major evolutionary event in ancestral Old World primates. *J. Human Evolution* 29:433-42.

Galili U & Matta KL. (1996) Inhibition of anti-Gal IgG binding to porcine endothelial cells by synthetic oligosaccharides. *Transplantation* 62: 256-62.

Galili U & Swanson K. (1991) Gene sequences suggest inactivation of α1,3 galactosyltransferase in catarrhines after the divergence of apes from monkeys. *Proc. Natl. Acad. Sci. USA* 88:7401-4.

Galili U, Rachmilewitz EA, Peleg A & Flechner I. (1984) A unique natural human IgG antibody with anti-α-galactosyl specificity. *J. Exp. Med.* 160:1519-31.

Galili U, Anaraki F, Thall A, Hill-Black C & Radic M. (1993) One percent of circulating B lymphocytes are capable of producing the natural anti-Gal antibody. *Blood*, 82: 2485-93.

Galili U, Buehler J, Shohet SB & Macher BA. (1987a) The human natural anti-Gal IgG. III. The subtlety of immune tolerance in man as demonstrated by crossreactivity between natural anti-Gal and anti-B antibodies. *J. Exp. Med.* 165:693-704.

Galili U, Chen, ZC, Tanemura M, Seregina T & Link CL. (2001) Induced Ab Response In Xenograft Recipients. *GRAFT* 4: 32-35.

Galili U, Clark MR, Shohet SB, Buehler J & Macher BA. (1987b) Evolutionary relationship between the anti-Gal antibody and the Gal-α1-3Gal epitope in primates. *Proc. Natl. Acad. Sci USA* 84:1369-73.

Galili U, LaTemple DC, Walgenbach AW & Stone KR (1997) Porcine and bovine cartilage transplants in cynomolgus monkey: II. Changes in anti-Gal response during chronic rejection. *Transplantation*, 63:646-651.

Galili U, Macher BA, Buehler J & Shohet SB. (1985) Human natural anti-α-galactosyl IgG. II. The specific recognition of α(1-3)-linked galactose residues. *J. Exp. Med.* 162:573-82.

Galili U, Mandrell RE, Hamadeh RM, Shohet SB & Griffis JM. (1988a) Interaction between human natural anti-α-galactosyl immunoglobulin G and bacteria of the human flora. *Infect. Immun.* 56, 1730-37.

Galili U, Shohet SB, Kobrin E, Stults CLM & Macher BA. (1988b) Man, apes, and Old World monkeys differ from other mammals in the expression of α-galactosyl epitopes on nucleated cells. *J. Biol. Chem.* 263:17755-62.

Galili U, Tibell A, Samuelsson B, Rydberg L & Groth CG. (1995) Increased anti-Gal activity in diabetic patients transplanted with fetal porcine islet cell clusters. *Transplantation*, 59: 1549-56.

Galili U. (1993) Interaction of the natural anti-Gal antibody with α-galactosyl epitopes: A major obstacle for xenotransplantation in humans. *Immunol Today* 14:480-82.

Galili U. (2004) Immune response, accommodation and tolerance to transplantation carbohydrate antigens. *Transplantation* 78: 1093-1098.

Good, AH, Cooper DCK, Malcolm AJ, Ippolito RM, Koren E, Neethling FA, Ye Y, Zuhdi N & Lamontage LR. (1992) Identification of carbohydrate structures which bind human anti-porcine antibodies: implication for discordant xenografting in man. *Transplant. Proc.* 24: 559-562.

Griesemer A, Liang F, Hirakata A, Hirsh E, Lo D, Okumi M, Sykes M, Yamada K, Huang CA & Sachs DH. (2010) Occurrence of specific humoral non-responsiveness to swine antigens following administration of GalT-KO bone marrow to baboons. *Xenotransplantation*. 17:300-12.

Griesemer AD, Hirakata A, Shimizu A, Moran S, Tena A, Iwaki H, Ishikawa Y, Schule P, Arn JS, Robson SC, Fishman JA, Sykes M, Sachs DH & Yamada K. (2009) Results of gal-knockout porcine thymokidney xenografts. *Am J Transplant*. 9:2669-78.

Groth CG, Korsgren O, Tibell A, Tollerman J, Möller E, Bolinder J, Ostman J, Reinholt FP, Hellerstrom C & Andersson A. (1994) Transplantation of fetal porcine pancreas to diabetic patients: biochemical and histological evidence for graft survival. *Lancet* 344:1402-4.

Hamadeh RM, Galili U, Zhou P & Griffis JM. (1995) Human secretions contain IgA, IgG and IgM anti-Gal (anti-α-galactosyl) antibodies. *Clin. Diagnos. Lab. Immunol.* 2:125-131.

Henion TR, Macher BA, Anaraki F & Galili U. (1994) Defining the minimal size of catalytically active primate α1,3galactosyltransferase: Structure function studies on the recombinant truncated enzyme. *Glycobiology* 4; 193-201.

Hisashi Y, Yamada K, Kuwaki K, Tseng YL, Dor FJ, Houser SL, Robson SC, Schuurman HJ, Cooper DK, Sachs DH, Colvin RB & Shimizu A. (2008) Rejection of cardiac xenografts transplanted from a1,3-galactosyltransferase gene-knockout (GalT-KO) pigs to baboons. *Am J Transplant*. 8:2516-26.

Joziasse DH, Shaper JH, Jabs EW, Shaper NL. (1991) Characterization of an α1-3-galactosyltransferase homologue on human chromosome 12 that is organized as a processed pseudogene, *J Biol Chem.* 15:266(11):6991-8

Koike C, Fung JJ, Geller DA, Kannagi R, Libert T, Luppi P, Nakashima I, Profozich J, Rudert W, Sharma SB, Starzl TE & Trucco M. (2002) Molecular Basis of Evolutionary Loss of the α1,3-Galactosyltransferase Gene in Higher Primates. *J. Biol. Chem.* 277:10114-20.

Kolber-Simonds D, Lai L, Watt SR, Denaro M, Arn S, Augenstein ML, Betthauser J, Carter DB, Greenstein JL, Hao Y, Im GS, Liu Z, Mell GD, Murphy CN, Park KW, Rieke A, Ryan DJ, Sachs DH, Forsberg EJ, Prather RS & Hawley RJ. (2004) Production of α1,3-galactosyltransferase null pigs by means of nuclear transfer with fibroblasts bearing loss of heterozygosity mutations. *Proc Natl Acad Sci U S A*.101:7335–40.

Korsgren O, Sandler S, Landström AS, Jansson L & Andersson A. (1988) Large-scale production of fetal porcine pancreatic isletlike cell clusters. An experimental tool for studies of islet cell differentiation and xenotransplantation. *Transplantation* 45: 509-14.

Kozlowski T, Ierino F, Lambrigts D, Foley A, Andrews D, Awwad M, Monroy R, Cosimi AB, Cooper DKC & Sachs DH. (1998) Depletion of anti-Galα1-3Gal antibody in baboons by specific α-Gal immunoaffinity columns. *Xenotransplantation* 5:122-31.

Kuwaki K, Tseng YL, Dor FJ, Shimizu A, Houser SL, Sanderson TM, Lancos CJ, Prabharasuth DD, Cheng J, Moran K, Hisashi Y, Mueller N, Yamada K, Greenstein JL, Hawley RJ, Patience C, Awwad M, Fishman JA, Robson SC, Schuurman HJ, Sachs DH & Cooper

DK. (2005) Heart transplantation in baboons using α1,3-galactosyltransferase gene-knockout pigs as donors: initial experience. *Nat Med.* 11:29-31.

Lam TT, Paniagua R, Shivaram G, Schuurman HJ, Borie DC & Morris RE. (2004) Anti-non-Gal porcine endothelial cell antibodies in acute humoral xenograft rejection of hDAF-transgenic porcine hearts in cynomolgus monkeys. *Xenotransplantation.* 11:531-35.

Larsen RD, Rivera-Marrero CA, Ernst LK, Cummings RD & Lowe JB. (1990) Frameshift and nonsense mutations in a human genomic sequence homologous to a murine UDP-Galβ-D-Gal(1,4)-D-GlcNAc α(1,3) galactosyltransferase cDNA. *J. Biol. Chem.* 265:7055-61.

Link CJ Jr, Moorman D, Seregina T, Levy JP & Schabold KJ. (1996) A phase I trial of in vivo gene therapy with the herpes simplex thymidine kinase/ganciclovir system for the treatment of refractory or recurrent ovarian cancer. *Hum. Gene Ther.* 7: 1161-79.

McGregor CG, Carpentier A, Lila N, Logan JS & Byrne GW. (2011) Cardiac xenotransplantation technology provides materials for improved bioprosthetic heart valves. *J Thorac Cardiovasc Surg.* 141:269-75.

McMorrow IM, Comrack CA, Sachs DH & DerSimonian H. (1997) Heterogeneity of human anti-pig natural antibodies cross-reactive with the Gal(α1,3)Galactose epitope. *Transplantation* 64: 501–510.

Miwa Y, Kobayashi T, Nagasaka T, Liu D, Yu M, Yokoyama I, Suzuki A, Nakao A. Are N-glycolylneuraminic acid (Hanganutziu-Deicher) antigens important in pig-to-human xenotransplantation? *Xenotransplantation* 2004; 11: 247-53.

Mohiuddin M, Ogawa H, Yin D & Galili U. (2003) Tolerance induction to a mammalian blood group like carbohydrate antigen by syngeneic lymphocytes expressing the antigen.: II. Tolerance induction on memory B cells. *Blood,* 102: 229-236.

Nemazee D, Kouskoff V, Hertz M, Lang J, Melamed D, Pape K & Retter M.l. (2000) B-cell-receptor- dependent positive and negative selection in immature B cells. *Curr Top Microbiol Immunol.;* 245: 57-71.

Ogawa H, & Galili U. (2006) Profiling terminal N-acetyllactoamines of glycans on mammalian cells by an immuno-enzymatic assay. *Glycoconjugate* J. 23: 663-74.

Ogawa H, Yin D, Shen J & Galili U. (2003) Tolerance induction to a mammalian blood group like carbohydrate antigen by syngeneic lymphocytes expressing the antigen. *Blood* 101:2318-2320.

Phelps CJ, Koike C, Vaught TD, Boone J, Wells KD, Chen SH, Ball S, Specht SM, Polejaeva IA, Monahan JA, Jobst PM, Sharma SB, Lamborn AE, Garst AS, Moore M, Demetris AJ, Rudert WA, Bottino R, Bertera S, Trucco M, Starzl TE, Dai Y & Ayares DL. (2003) Production of α1,3-galactosyltransferase-deficient pigs. *Science.* 299:411-14.

Pilbeam D. The descent of hominoids and hominids. *Sci Am.* 250:84-96, 1984.

Sandel PC, Monroe JG. Negative selection of immature B cells by receptor editing or deletion is determined by site of antigen encounter. *Immunity* 1999; 10: 289-99.

Sandrin M, Vaughan HA, Dabkowski PL & McKenzi IFC. (1993) Anti-pig IgM Abs in human serum react predominantly with Galα1-3Gal epitopes. *Proc. Natl. Acad. Sci. USA* 90:11391-95.

Simon PM, Neethling FA, Taniguchi S, Goode PL, Zopf D, Hancock WW & Cooper DK. (1998) Intravenous infusion of Galα1-3Gal oligosaccharides in baboon delays hyperacute rejection of porcine heart xenografts. *Transplantation* 56: 346-53.

Springer GF, Horton RE. (1969) Blood group isoantibody stimulation in man by feeding blood group-active bacteria. *J Clin Invest.* 48:1280-91.

Stone KR, Abdel-Motal U, Walgenbach AW, Turek TJ & Galili U. (2007) Replacement of human anterior cruciate ligament with pig ligament: a model for anti-non gal antibody response in long-term xenotransplantation. *Transplantation,* 83: 211-219.

Takahagi Y, Fujimura T, Miyagawa S, Nagashima H, Shigehisa T, Shirakura R, Murakami H. (2005) Production of α1,3-galactosyltransferase gene knockout pigs expressing both human decay-accelerating factor and N-acetylglucosaminyltransferase III. *Mol Reprod Dev.* 71:331-8.

Tanemura M, Yin D, Chong AS & Galili U. (2000) Differential immune responses to α-gal epitopes on xenografts and allografts: implications for accommodation in xenotransplantation. *J. Clin. Invest.* 105:301-10.

Taylor RE, Gregg CJ, Padler-Karavani V, Ghaderi D, Yu H, Huang S, Sorensen RU, Chen X, Inostroza J, Nizet V & Varki A. (2010) Novel mechanism for the generation of human xeno-autoantibodies against the nonhuman sialic acid N-glycolylneuraminic acid. *J Exp Med.* 207:1637-46.

Thall A, Etienne-Decerf J, Winand R & Galili U. (1991) The α-galactosyl epitope on mammalian thyroid cells. *Acta Endocrin.* 124:692-99.

Tseng YL, Kuwaki K, Dor FJ, Shimizu A, Houser S, Hisashi Y, Yamada K, Robson SC, Awwad M, Schuurman HJ, Sachs DH, & Cooper DK. (2005) α1,3-Galactosyltransferase gene-knockout pig heart transplantation in baboons with survival approaching 6 months. *Transplantation.* 80:1493-500.

Wang L, Radic MZ & Galili U. (1995) Human anti-Gal heavy chain genes. Preferential use of VH3 and the presence of somatic mutations. *J. Immunol.* 155:1276-85.

Watier H, Guillaumin J-M, Vallee I, Thibault G, Gruel Y, Lebranchu Y & Bardos P. (1996) Human NK cell-mediated direct and IgG dependent cytotoxicity against xenogeneic porcine endothelial cells. *Transplant. Immunol.* 4:293-99.

Wilson AC & Sarich VM. (1969) A molecular time scale for human evolution. *Proc Natl Acad Sci U S A.* 63:1088-93.

Xu T, Lorf T, Sablinski T, Gianello P, Bailin M, Monroy R, Kozlowski T, Cooper DK & Sachs DH. (1998) Removal of anti-porcine natural antibodies from human and nonhuman primate plasma in vitro and in vivo by a Galα1-3Galβ1-4Glc-R immunoaffinity column. *Transplantation* 65:172-79.

Yamada K, Yazawa K, Shimizu A, Iwanaga T, Hisashi Y, Nuhn M, O'Malley P, Nobori S, Vagefi PA, Patience C, Fishman J, Cooper DK, Hawley RJ, Greenstein J, Schuurman HJ, Awwad M, Sykes M & Sachs DH. (2005) Marked prolongation of porcine renal xenograft survival in baboons through the use of α1,3-galactosyltransferase gene-knockout donors and the cotransplantation of vascularized thymic tissue. *Nat Med.* 11:32-34.

Yeh P, Ezzelarab M, Bovin N, Hara H, Long C, Tomiyama K, Sun F, Ayares D, Awwad M & Cooper DK. (2010) Investigation of potential carbohydrate antigen targets for human and baboon antibodies. *Xenotransplantation.* 17:197-206.

Yu PB, Parker W, Everett ML, Fox IJ & Platt JL. (1999) Immunochemical properties of anti-Galα1-3Gal antibodies after sensitization with xenogeneic tissues. *J Clin. Immunol.* 19: 116-26.

Zhu A & Hurst R. (2002) Anti-N-glycolylneuraminic acid antibodies identified in healthy human serum. *Xenotransplantation.* 9:376-81.

2

Piscine Islet Xenotransplantation

James R. Wright, Jr.
University of Calgary Department of Pathology and Laboratory Medicine & Calgary Laboratory Services Canada

1. Introduction

In type I diabetes mellitus, the insulin-producing β-cells have been destroyed by an autoimmune process and, thus, these patients are dependent upon daily insulin injections to sustain life; however, insulin injections are not a cure in that most patients eventually develop long-term complications due to imprecise control of blood glucose levels. Although one or more insulin injections, carefully coordinated with precise dietary and exercise regimens, can improve glycemic control, there is still considerable fluctuation of blood sugar levels throughout the day. Furthermore, excessive insulin administration can cause hypoglycaemia, coma, and brain damage. Insulin administration simply cannot provide the degree of glycemic control provided by the intact pancreatic islet. Normal islets function like thermostats except that they regulate blood glucose levels rather than temperature; islets recognize high or low blood glucose levels and respond by increasing or decreasing insulin secretion on a moment by moment basis, thus providing precise glycemic control throughout the day. There is considerable evidence that precise control of blood glucose levels will prevent the chronic complications of diabetes (Wolffenbuttel, 1993), and this is the primary rationale supporting pancreatic islet transplantation.

Islet allotransplantation could allow for an actual "cure" for type I, and possibly also many patients with type II, diabetes; however, there are several perplexing problems (CITR Research Group, 2009). First of all, although considerable progress has been made with immunosuppressive regimens to promote islet allograft survival, long-term insulin independence occurs in less than 25% of patients; furthermore, there are potential complications associated with long-term immunosuppression. Therefore, islet allotransplantation is usually limited to type I diabetic patients who have difficulty controlling glycemic levels with insulin therapy and who have frequent hypoglycemic episodes. Second, in human (and mammalian) pancreases, islets comprise only 1-2% of the pancreas by volume and are scattered throughout. Isolating human islets is not an exact science. Currently, it often requires several human donor pancreases to obtain sufficient islets for a single transplant and the costs associated with each islet isolation procedure are huge. Third, and most importantly, there are simply an inadequate number of suitable human cadaveric donors. There are currently several million type 1 diabetic patients in North America and, each year, there are several tens of thousands of new cases; in stark contrast, there are less than ten thousand suitable donors per year. Thus, the supply of islets is a limiting factor that would likely prevent widespread application of clinical islet allotransplantation.

Clinical islet xenotransplantation, which could result in a potentially unlimited supply of donor islets, could be an attractive alternative. However, xenotransplantation creates an entirely new set of issues including: (1) selection of an appropriate donor species, (2) xenograft rejection, (3) risk of xenozoonotic disease transmission, (4) animal rights issues, (5) complicated ethical issues pertaining to the rights of recipients, close contacts, and society as a whole, (6) difficult institutional, national, and international regulatory issues, (7) very high potential costs, and (8) whether precious healthcare dollars could be better spent, especially in countries like Canada with public supported healthcare systems (Wright et al., 2004). This chapter will focus primarily on the selection of an appropriate donor but will touch on many of these other issues in passing.

2. Experimental islet xenotransplantation using tilapia donors

Unlike mammalians which have very large numbers of very small (microscopic) islets scattered amongst the exocrine pancreas (and comprising only 1-2% of its total volume), many teleost (i.e., bony) fish have small numbers of very large islets as discrete islet organs called Brockmann bodies. Because these large islets are macroscopically visible and easy to harvest, they actually played an important role in the discovery of insulin and have even been used sporadically over the past 90 years as a source of insulin for clinical treatment of diabetic patients (Wright, 2002a; Wright, 2002b).

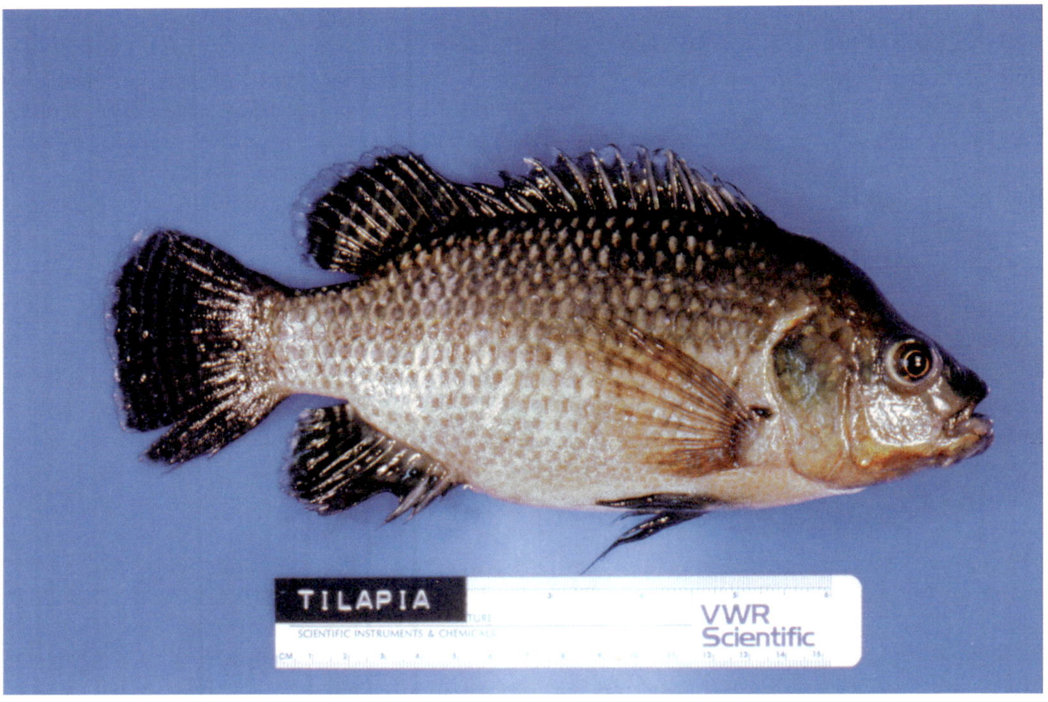

Fig. 1. The Nile Tilapia is a popular food world-wide. It is often produced in large aquaculture systems. A "market size" tilapia weighs about 700-800 grams. The maximum size, in our hands, is about 5kg (0.5 meter in length). Most of our transplant work is done with tilapia weighing between 500-1,200gm.

We have used tilapia (*Oreochromis niloticus;* figure 1), a large, commercially important warm water teleost species, as a source of islets for xenotransplantation research since 1992 (Wright, 1992). We and others have shown that tilapia islets transplanted under the kidney capsules of streptozotocin-diabetic athymic nude mice provide long-term normoglycemia and mammalian-like glucose tolerance profiles (Wright et al., 1992; Morsiani et al., 1995; Leventhal et al, 2004). When transplanted into mice with a normal immune system, tilapia islet grafts are functionally and histologically rejected in 7-8 days (Wright et al., 1994) and graft rejection is characterized by massive infiltration of macrophages, eosinophils, and T-cells (Wright et al., 1997). In general, tilapia islet xenograft rejection is temporally and mechanistically similar to rejection of pig or human islets (Dickson et al., 2003).

2.1 Harvesting and transplanting tilapia brockmann bodies

Harvesting tilapia islets is very simple; unlike mammalian islets, there is no need for inflating pancreatic ducts with expensive blends of special collagenases followed by complicated, time-consuming, and fickle islet isolation procedures. As shown in figure 2, Tilapia Brockmann bodies are scattered within the adipose tissue surrounding the common bile duct in a triangular region bounded anteriorly by the edge of the liver, superiorly by the stomach, and inferiorly by the spleen and gall bladder (i.e., "the Brockmann body region").

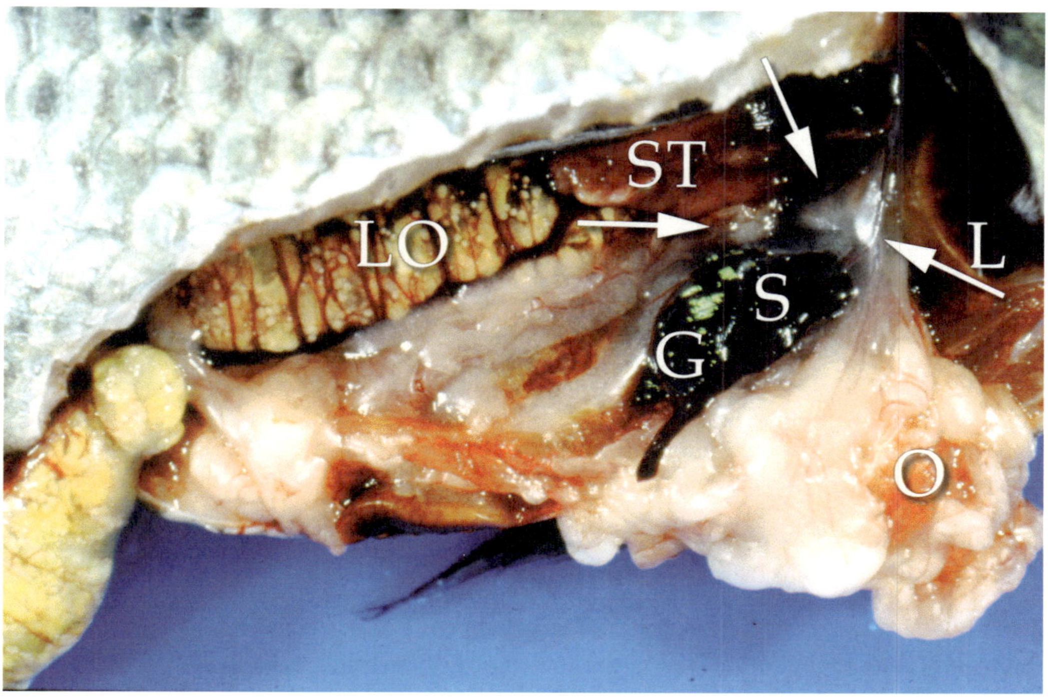

Fig. 2. Dissection of female tilapia with the right ovary and omentum (O) reflected downward reveals the roughly triangular Brockmann body region (outlined by arrows) surrounded by the liver (L), stomach (ST), and spleen (S) and gall bladder (G). LO=left ovary. Reprinted with permission from Yang H, Wright JR Jr. 1995. A method for mass harvesting islets (Brockmann bodies) from teleost fish. Cell Transplantation 4, pp. (621-628).

The larger islets can be removed simply by excising the entire "region" (figure 3 & figure 4), placing it in a plastic petri dish with Hank's Balanced Salt Solution, and microdissecting them from the adipose tissue while visualizing them with a dissecting microscope (Wright, 1994). This method works fine but would be inefficient if doing more than a few transplants as it is slow and misses the smaller islets. Alternatively, the islets can be enzymatically mass-harvested by removing regions from multiple fish simultaneously, placing them in a tube with a type II collagenase (normally used to harvest adipocytes) solution, and then placing the tube in a 37^{0}C shaker water bath for 10 minutes; when the incubation period is over, the digestion is stopped by adding cold Hank's, causing the fat cells to float to the top of the tube and islets to remain as a pellet (Yang & Wright, 1995).

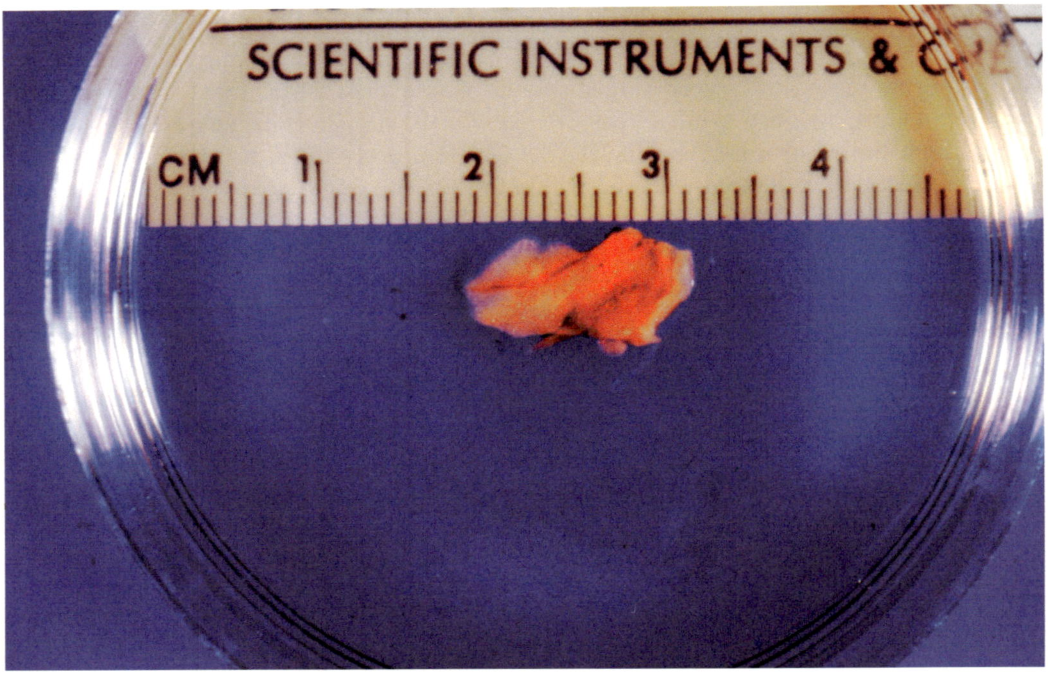

Fig. 3. Excised Brockmann body "region" free floating in Hanks balanced solution salt solution. Reprinted with permission from Yang H, Wright JR Jr. 1995. A method for mass harvesting islets (Brockmann bodies) from teleost fish. Cell Transplantation 4, pp. (621-628).

It should be noted that in large tilapia, some Brockmann bodies can measure up to 5 mm in maximum dimension [n.b., tilapia produce new islets and their older islets grow throughout their lifespan and so there is a tremendous range in islet size (Morrison et al., 2004)]. For our transplantation work, all large islets are broken up into smaller "mammalian islet" sized fragments (Yang et al., 1997a). After overnight culture, these fragmented islets "round up" and then take on the appearance of mammalian islets. Fragmented islets can then be transplanted immediately, cultured under various conditions (Wright & Kearns, 1995), or cryopreserved in liquid nitrogen (O'Hali et al., 1997). Fragmentation does not affect the cellular composition or function of the islets because the large islets are comprised of repetitive units similar to smaller islets (Yang et al., 1999a). There is a linear relationship between fish body weight and the number of islet endocrine cells (Dickson et al., 1998); therefore, the sum of the body weights of multiple donor fish can be used to predict the total islet cell mass as well as the number of transplants that can be performed (Wright et al., 2004).

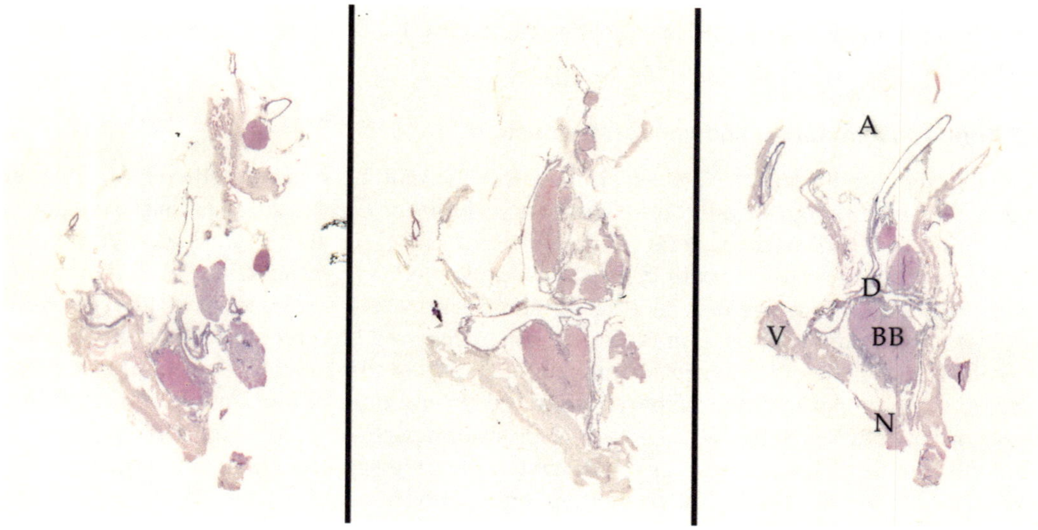

Fig. 4. Whole mount produced by processing an entire Brockmann body region for histology. Sections were cut at three different levels through the block to provide a three-dimensional view. Sections were stained with hematoxylin and eosin. The regions are composed of adipose tissue (A), bile and pancreatic ducts (D), blood vessels (V), nerve (N), and Brockmann bodies (BB). Twelve Brockmann bodies can be identified in the center frame. Reprinted with permission from Yang H, Wright JR Jr. 1995. A method for mass harvesting islets (Brockmann bodies) from teleost fish. Cell Transplantation 4, pp. (621-628).

In rodents, unencapsulated tilapia islets can be transplanted under the kidney capsule (Yang et al., 1997a), via the portal vein (Al-Jazaeri et al., 2005), or into the non-cryptorchid testes (Coddington et al., 1997). When islets are transplanted into any of these sites, the grafts undergo neovascularisation (i.e., recipient capillaries grow into the grafts). This is one of the features that makes islet transplantation different from whole organ transplantation, in which immediate direct vascular anastomoses are performed. Because Brockmann bodies are discrete and separate from the exocrine pancreas, it is also possible to transplant them as immediately vascularised grafts by microvascular surgical techniques (Yu et al., 2003), creating the unique ability to compare these grafts as either neovascularized cell transplants or directly vascularised organ grafts. This is particularly interesting in the context that tilapia cells are too primitive to express α(1,3) gal, an antigen expressed on mammalian cells (except human and Old World apes), that is responsible for hyperacute rejection of whole organ xenografts in man (Leventhal et al., 2004). Fish islets are also unique in that they can be transplanted into the non-cryptorchid testis; in contrast, mammalian islets only function if transplanted into the cryptorchid testis. The reason for this difference is that the fish are poikilotherms and their islets are fully functional at a wider range of body temperatures whereas mammalian islets require 37°C. Tilapia islets are very well-suited for encapsulation (see below).

For experimental studies in which rejection is based upon monitoring function (i.e., ability to lower blood glucose levels), tilapia islets have a major advantage compared to either fetal or neonatal porcine islets, as the latter do not become functional until they have matured after transplantation. Tilapia islets, like adult pig islets, function immediately after transplantation.

2.2 Xenotransplantation and xenograft rejection

Initially, we used tilapia islets as an inexpensive tool to screen methods directed at preventing islet xenograft rejection. The vast majority of early studies on islet xenografts were done with the concordant rat-to-mouse model and these studies implied that the islet xenograft rejection process could be easily circumvented (Wright & Yang, 1997). However, when methods that prevented islet xenograft rejection between concordant species were applied to discordant species combinations, most conferred little real protection. Intuitively, it seemed that it would be hard to imagine any species combination that would be more discordant than fish-to-mammal by virtue of the several hundred million years separating, these orders phylogenetically. The results of studies testing various modalities for their ability to prevent islet xenograft rejection have been reviewed elsewhere but, in general, we found that methods directed at decreasing graft immunogenicity prior to transplantation were ineffective but that chronic high dose immunosuppression was reasonably effective at prolonging islet xenograft survival(Wright & Yang, 1997; Wright & Pohajdak, 2001); however, the latter could precipitate post-transplant lymphoproliferative disorder (Yang et al., 2002b). We also developed a heterotopic heart transplant model to prove that xenotransplantation from tilapia to rodent was actually discordant (Yu & Wright, 1999).

We also used the tilapia-to-mouse model to study the mechanism of xenograft rejection. Generally speaking, the mechanism of rejection of tilapia islets is highly CD4 dependent and appears to be no different than the rejection of pig islets (Dickson et al., 2003). Immune destruction of encapsulated tilapia islets (see below) in spontaneously diabetic NOD mice is also CD4 dependent (Xu et al., 2005).

2.3 Xenotransplantation with encapsulation

Encapsulation devices are small semi-permeable chambers in which islets can be placed prior to transplantation and which are designed to protect the islet grafts from the host's immune system (de Vos et al., 2010; Vaithilingam & Tuch, 2011). These devices are generally divided into macroencapsulation and microencapsulation devices. Both achieve immunoprotection by creating a barrier with "pore" sizes small enough to prevent leukocytes and antibodies from damaging the graft but large enough for oxygen, insulin, glucose and nutrients to pass freely. Encapsulation devices, in general, have a number of associated problems including: (1) none are entirely biocompatible, (2) hypoxia causes graft attrition , (3) device durability issues, (4) pores can shed antigen precipitating inflammation, fibroplasia, and humoral sensitization, (5) cytokines can enter the pores, (6) devices must be replaced or refilled periodically, and (7) devices increase total graft bulk.

Relative to mammalian islets, tilapia islets are highly resistant to hypoxia (Wright et al., 1998b) making them ideal for incorporation into transplantable encapsulation devices (Yang & Wright, 2002a). We have previously shown that encapsulation markedly prolongs piscine islet xenograft survival in small animal recipients (Yang et al., 1997) and that co-encapsulation with allogenic or xenogeneic Sertoli cells further prolongs graft survival (Yang & Wright, 1999). Interestingly, the protective effect of Sertoli cells is not mediated by their Fas-ligand expression as Fas-L deficient Sertoli cells still confer protection (Yang et al., 2002a).

Dionne et al. (1994) have described the "idealized" islet for incorporation into encapsulation devices as follows. "The ideal tissue has a high insulin output, is correctly regulated by glucose and other secretogogues, has low metabolic demand, and is capable of functioning for extended periods without replacement. In addition, the cells must be procurable in high yield at reasonable cost with protocol meeting FDA standards (Dionne et al., 1994). In general, tilapia islets meet these criteria. However, to this definition, we would also add the need for a human insulin-like structure (see below).

3. Potential clinical islet xenotransplantation using tilapia donors

Because tilapia islets appear physiologically capable of providing long-term normoglycemia and mammalian-like glucose tolerance profiles, we believe that they could play a future role in clinical islet xenotransplantation. However, there are some significant issues.

First of all, islets are not simply sources of insulin. Islets are comprised of multiple cell types which produce other hormones. In the context of a xenograft, it occurred to us that some of these foreign peptides might either have undesirable biological activity or, even if these other foreign peptides were non-functional, they might serve as antigens and promote antibody reactions as well as immune complex diseases.

Second, little is known about how fish islets maintain normoglycemia. Before one could consider transplanting fish islets into humans, tilapia β-cell physiology would need to be examined.

Third, although it is known that fish insulins are functional in humans (Wright, 2002a; Wright, 2002b), their amino acid sequences usually differ considerably from that of human insulin and their relative biological activities in man are variable. Tilapia insulin structure differs from human insulin by a total of 17 amino acids (Nguyen et al., 1995), whereas, in contrast, porcine insulin differs at only the 30th amino acid on the B-chain.

Fourth, although it was not known when we began this research, it is now believed that all fish possess two non-allelic insulin genes. Little is known about the Insulin-2 gene in tilapia or other fish.

3.1 Other islet peptides

Like mammalian islets, tilapia Brockmann bodies are mostly comprised of insulin-producing β-cells, glucagon-producing α-cells, and somatostatin (SST)-producing δ-cells. However, there are some fundamental differences. First of all, the fourth primary peptide in mammalian islets is Pancreatic Polypeptide while in tilapia it is Peptide-YY; both typically represent 1-2% of the islet cells and will not be further discussed here. Second, fish islets have two different types of δ-cells, one producing the 14 amino acid SST-1 (n.b., the sequence of this peptide is identical in all vertebrates) and the other a "large" SST, the product of the preproSST-II gene (either not present or not expressed in mammals). Third, the percentages of the different cell types in mammals and tilapia differ greatly. In mammals, the insulin-producing β-cells predominate (~70%), glucagon-producing α-cells represent ~20%, and SST-producing δ-cells comprise <10%; in tilapia, the percentage of β, α, δ−1, and δ-2 cells are 42.3%, 11.5%, 21.8%, and 23.1% (Yang et al., 1999a). Fourth, the glucagon-producing α-cells in fish simultaneous produce glucagon-like peptide (GLP)-1; mammals, in contrast, produce two different GLPs, GLP-1 and GLP-2, and GLP-1 is produced in the intestinal L-cells, while fish make only GLP-1, and it is produced only in the islet α-cells. Fifth, in mammals, most islets are composed of a central β-cell core and the non-β-cells are at the periphery of the islet; in contrast each tilapia Brockmann body, which is much larger than mammalian islet, is comprised of many repetitive units containing a central core of β-cells encased by a thin layer of SST-1 δ-cells which are surrounded by SST-2 δ-cells and scattered α-cells (Yang et al., 1999a). Because of this highly repetitive nature, Brockmann bodies fragmented for transplantation contain all cell types.

These differences create several interesting scenarios related to xenotransplantation. First of all, in the context of the two different SSTs, SST-1 is 100% homologous with all mammalian SSTs, and, thus, should be biologically active while the second large SST would be biologically irrelevant and likely antigenic and could potentially precipitate immune complex disease. However, after xenotransplantation into streptozotocin-diabetic nude mice, the cells producing this peptide, the δ-2-cells, decreased from roughly 25% of the cells in the islet graft to negligible numbers in less than 2 months, apparently due to apoptosis secondary to the lack of any piscine trophic stimulation after xenotransplantation into a mammalian environment (Morrison et al., 2003b). Equally interesting was the observation that the percentage of the various endocrine cell types in the grafts became increasingly mammalian-like as time passed (Morrison et al., 2003b). One further observation was that co-expression of GLP-1 and glucagon persisted throughout the study. This is intriguing as GLP-1 is known to promote improved glucose homeostasis and β-cell neogenesis, which could be an advantageous by-product of fish islet xenotransplantation.

3.2 Glucose homeostasis and β–cell function in tilapia

Until recently, little was known about glucose homeostasis in fish. This is probably not surprising as there are very few fish species in which glucose is a significant component of their natural diets. In fact, it was generally believed that fish islets were not particularly glucose responsive (Wright et al., 2000). However, a simple xenotransplantation study using tilapia islets disproved this. In this study, glucose tolerance tests were performed in intact fish and it took them roughly 3 days to dispose of glucose loads, thus demonstrating extreme glucose intolerance (as had been shown previously in other fish species); however, when the tilapia islets were harvested from donor fish and engrafted under the kidney capsule of streptozotocin-diabetic nude mice, these same islets disposed of an equivalent glucose load in less than 30 minutes, suggesting that insulin secretion by tilapia islets was highly glucose-responsive but that the reason tilapia (and presumably other fish) were glucose intolerant was because of an extreme peripheral resistance to the glucostatic effects of insulin (Wright et al., 1998a). More recently, we have confirmed the glucose responsiveness of tilapia islets *in vitro* and have dissected the regulation of insulin gene expression and insulin production in tilapia islets (Hrytsenko et al., 2008). Interestingly, we also found insulin gene expression in the tilapia brain and pituitary (Hrytsenko et al., 2007).

Like in mammalian islets, the "glucose sensor" in the tilapia β-cell is glucokinase (Joy, 2002). However, the glucose sensor must partner with a glucose transporter and we are less certain as to the primary glucose transporter in the tilapia β-cell (Alexander et al., 2006; Hrytsenko et al., 2010). In rodent islets, GLUT-2 is the primary glucose transporter but in human islets it is GLUT-1. We have demonstrated high levels of expression of both transporters in tilapia Brockmann bodies; however, circumstantial evidence leads us to favor GLUT-1. Streptozotocin and alloxan are highly toxic to rodent β-cells and induce severe diabetes; both are known to enter the β-cell via GLUT-2 rather than GLUT-1; human β-cells, which preferentially utilize GLUT-1, are highly resistant to both drugs. Tilapia β-cells, like human β-cells, are resistant to the diabetogenic effects of streptozotocin and alloxan (Wright et al., 1999; Yang & Wright, 2002b; Xu et al., 2004).

Alexander et al. (2006) have reviewed many other aspects of tilapia islet physiology. The readers are referred to this review for a more detailed analysis.

3.3 Tilapia insulin structure and transgenic tilapia expressing a humanized insulin gene

Although tilapia islets provide many advantages relative to mammalian islets, the tilapia insulin structure differs from human insulin structure by 17 amino acids and we felt that this would likely preclude their clinical use. Therefore, we decided to make and patent transgenic tilapia expressing a "humanized" tilapia insulin gene (Wright & Pohajdak, 2000; Wright & Pohajdak, 2002). This was accomplished by cloning and sequencing the tilapia insulin gene (Mansour et al. 1998), modifying it by site directed mutagenesis changing only the codons representing the 17 amino acids that differed between human and tilapia insulin, and then microinjecting the "humanized" tilapia insulin transgene via the micropile into fertilized tilapia eggs (Pohajdak et al., 2004). Resulting offspring were simultaneously screened by PCR using tilapia insulin gene-specific primers and humanized tilapia insulin gene-specific primers. One founder, who was later shown to be a mosaic (Wright et al., 2008), demonstrated germ-line expression and passed the transgene on to some of his offspring. Positive offspring were segregated and grown to a size large enough to safely bleed and collect plasma for human insulin measurements. Some offspring with high levels of circulating human insulin were sacrificed for histology; figure 5 shows the presence of human insulin-positive β-cells in a transgenic Brockmann body and absence of human insulin staining in β-cells from a wild-type tilapia Brockmann body. Figure 6 shows that islet architecture (i.e., distribution of other endocrine cell types) is unchanged in transgenic tilapia islets.

It should be noted, in order to maintain appropriate cleavage by the endopeptidases, the terminal amino acid on the B-chain was omitted and, therefore, our trangenics secrete [desThrB30] human insulin. In comparison, porcine insulin differs from human insulin by substitution of an Ala for the terminal Thr; whereas our transgenic human insulin is simply missing the terminal Thr.

Eventually, while battling government regulatory and other nightmares (Wright, 2006; Wright et al., 2012), we were able to breed these transgenic fish to homozygosity and have now demonstrated lifelong transgene expression (Hrytsenko et al., 2010; Hrytsenko et al., 2011). We hope to begin early pre-clinical transplantation studies soon.

(A)

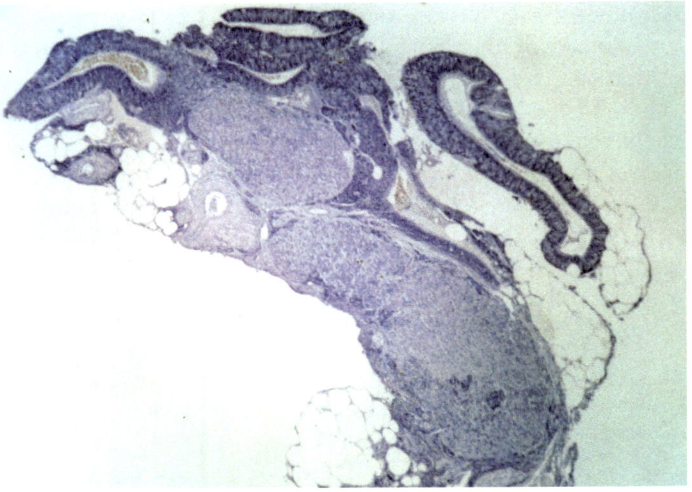

(B)

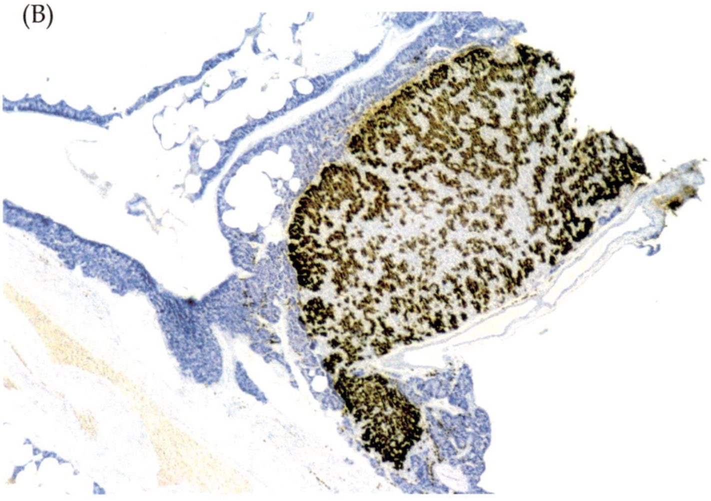

Fig. 5. Histologic sections of pancreatic islets from control (A) and transgenic (B) juvenile tilapia. Sections are stained for human insulin by immunoperoxidase. Note the clusters of immunopositive β-cells in the transgenic islets and the absence of staining in the control islets. Consistent results were obtained using several different commercially available monoclonal and polyclonal antibodies for human insulin. Reprinted with permission from Pohajdak B, Mansour M, Hrytsenko O, Conlon JM, Dymond C, & Wright JR Jr. 2004. Production of transgenic tilapia with Brockmann bodies secreting [desThrB30] human insulin. Transgenic Res. 13, 4, pp. (313-323).

Eventually, we believe that we will need to either knockout the native tilapia insulin gene or at least silence it. Methods for producing gene knockout fish are still in their infancy with almost all of the work in this field having been performed in zebrafish or Japanese medaka. In general, the process, like in mice, will likely involve creating ES cells from tilapia blastulas at the ~1000 cell stage, knocking out the native tilapia insulin gene *in vitro* through homologous recombination, and then microinjecting these ES-cells back into developing tilapia blastulas, screening for cutaneous chimerism, screening these chimeras for germ-line chimerism, and then breeding to homozygosity. Little of the work done in zebrafish and medaka is directly applicable and so we have done some of the preliminary work characterizing early embryogenesis in tilapia to facilitate these studies (Morrison et al., 2001; Morrison et al. 2003a) and have demonstrated the ability to make chimeras by microinjecting blastula cells (Wright et al., 2012).

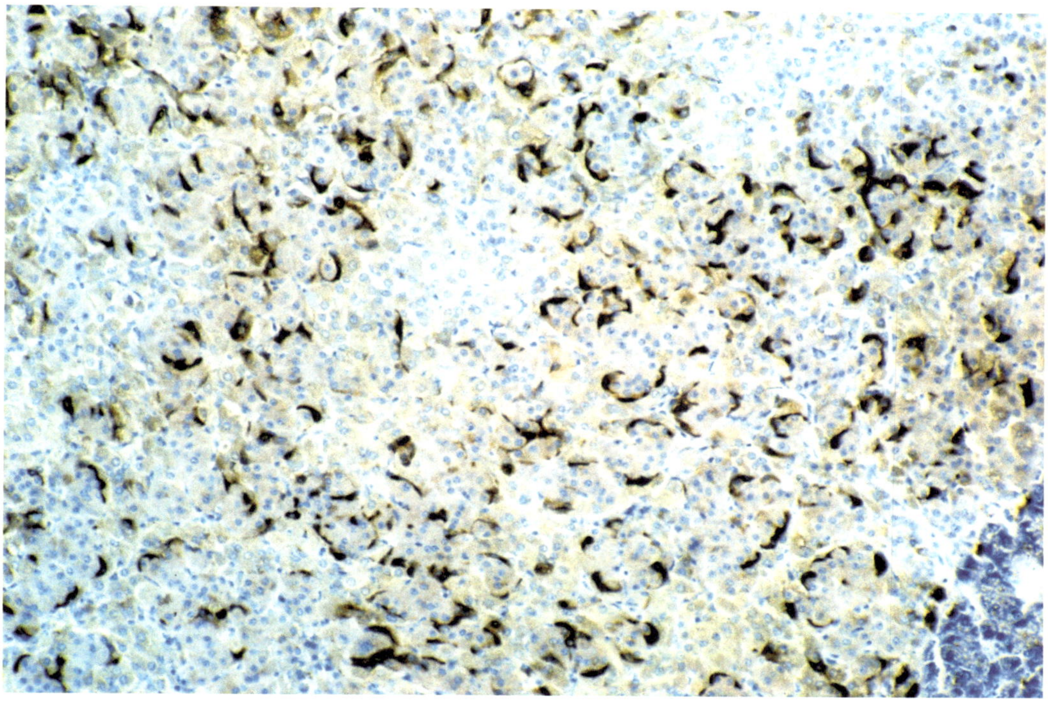

Fig. 6. Histologic sections of pancreatic islets from transgenic tilapia stained for human SST-1 by immunoperoxidase. Note the concave shape of individual and small groups of SST-1+ δ-cells. These cells directly encase clusters of β-cells and are surrounded by SST-2+ δ-cells (staining not shown here). The overall architecture of the Brockmann body is unchanged in transgenics.

3.4 Two non-allelic insulin genes

Recently, from studying genomic maps of zebrafish, medaka, and fugu (pufferfish), it has become apparent that ancestral fish underwent a genomic duplication several hundred million years ago and that these modern-day fish possess a second non-allelic insulin gene (Taylor et al., 2003). This may not be surprising as genome duplication appears to have played a major role in evolution as the "big leaps" cannot be explained by natural selection acting on necessary genes; big leaps required new gene loci with redundant function that could accumulate forbidden mutations (Conlon & Larhammar, 2005). Furthermore, such an insulin gene duplication would not be unique as it has long been known that rat and mouse islets express two non-allelic insulin genes (Lomedico et al., 1980) and there is even some evidence that the porcine insulin gene may be duplicated (Snel & Damgaard, 1980).

However, it critical to know whether tilapia have two non-allelic insulin genes and, if so, whether the second insulin gene is expressed and a product secreted as the transgenic tilapia that we produced by microinjecting a "humanized" tilapia insulin gene possess islets that simultaneously secrete both human insulin and tilapia insulin. Therefore, our plan is to knock out or silence the native tilapia insulin gene in these transgenics, resulting in donors with islets that secrete only human insulin. However, unless it has been deleted during evolution, it seemed highly probable that tilapia possess a second insulin gene and that, if it is expressed, this might adversely affect our ability to produce a donor strain with islets secreting only human insulin.

Therefore, degenerative primers were designed based upon the alignment of the available sequences for fish insulin 2 genes and we cloned most of the NTins2 (nile tilapia insulin 2) gene and studied tissue-specific expression. Analysis of the primary protein organization revealed that the precursor molecule consists of the four typical preproinsulin regions: signal peptide, B chain, C chain, and A chain; prohormone convertase processing sites were determined and the peptide appeared to be potentially biologically active (Hrytsenko, 2007).

Using qRT-PCR, we examined the levels of Insulin 2 gene expression in islets and other tissues and compared this with Insulin 1 gene and actin expression. Insulin 2 gene expression occurred in all tested tissues, except for adipose tissue, at exceedingly low levels, and the level of expression in tilapia islets was not significantly higher than in other tissues. This almost uniform pattern of insulin 2 expression resembles the expression pattern for house keeping genes, and is in contrast to the more tightly restricted β-cell-specific transcription of the insulin 1 gene. It is most likely that the NTins2 gene is transcribed at low levels in essentially all extrapancreatic tissues and its transcription is only slightly up-regulated in the pancreatic islets. Moreover, translation of the second insulin may actually be suppressed by the presence of a short reading frame upstream of the insulin initiation codon (Hrytsenko, 2007). Regardless, it seems unlikely that the insulin 2 product will need to be silenced in transgenic tilapia islets.

4. Conclusions

As documented above, tilapia islets have played a significant role in experimental islet xenotransplantation research. Advantages include ease of harvesting, total cost of procured islets, and the ability to transplant them into multiple body sites and have them function immediately after transplantation (not true for either fetal or neonatal pig islets); on the other hand, the major disadvantage is the need for specialized animal housing facilities, as aquatic facilities are not available at all research institutions. Transgenic tilapia islets expressing a humanized insulin gene may also play a role in future clinical islet xenotransplantation. We now have homozygous transgenics ready for pre-clinical testing.

We conservatively estimate, based upon animal husbandry and islet isolation costs, that production costs for transgenic tilapia islets should be at least 100-fold less expensive than porcine islets on a per clinical transplant basis (Wright et al., 2004). This advantage could greatly facilitate the widespread implementation of clinical islet xenotransplantation as a cure for type I diabetes.

5. Acknowledgment

Financial support has been provided by the Juvenile Diabetes Research Foundation, the University of Calgary Faculty of Medicine, and Calgary Laboratory Services.

6. References

Alexander E, Dooley KC, Pohajdak B, & Wright JR Jr. (2006). Things we've learned from tilapia islet xenotransplantation. *Gen. Com. Endocrinol.* 148, 2, pp. (125-131)

Al-Jazaeri A, Xu B-Y, Yang H, MacNeil D, Leventhal JR, & Wright JR Jr. (2005). Effect of glucose toxicity on intraportal tilapia islet xenotransplantation in nude mice. *Xenotransplantation* 12, pp. (189-196)

Coddington DA, Lawen JG, Yang H, O'Hali W, & Wright JR Jr. (1997). Xenotransplantation of fish islets into the non-cryptorchid testis. *Transplant. Proc.* 29, pp. (2083-2085)

Conlon JM & Larhammar D. (2005). The evolution of neuroendocrine peptides. *Gen. Comp. Endocrinol.* 142, pp. (53-59)

CITR Research Group. (2009). 2007 update on allogeneic islet transplantation from the Collaborative Islet Transplant Registry (CITR). *Cell Transplant.* 18, 7, pp. (753-767)

de Vos P, Spasojevic M, & Faas MM. (2010). Treatment of diabetes with encapsulated islets. *Adv Exp Med Biol.* 670, pp. (38-53)

Dickson B, Yang H, Pohajdak B, & Wright JR Jr. (1998). Quantification of tilapia islets: a direct relationship between islet cell number and body mass. *Transplant. Proc.* 30, pp. (621-622)

Dickson BC, Yang H, Savelkoul HFJ, Rowden G, van Rooijen N, & Wright JR Jr. (2003). Islet transplantation in the discordant tilapia-to-mouse model: a novel application of alginate microencapsulation in the study of xenograft rejection. *Transplantation* 75, pp. (599-606)

Dionne K, Scharp D, Lysaght M Hegre P, & Lacy P. (1994). Macroencapsulation of islets for the treatment of diabetes. In: *Lanza PR, Chick WL, eds. Pancreatic Islet Transplantation. Vol. 3. Immunoisolation of the Pancreatic Islets*, RG Landes Co., pp. (119-131), Austin

Hrytsenko O. (2007). Molecular characterization of the insulin genes in Nile tilapia (*Oreochromis niloticus*). PhD Dissertation, Dalhousie University, Halifax, Nova Scotia, Canada

Hrytsenko O, Pohajdak B, & Wright JR Jr. (2010). Production of transgenic tilapia homozygous for a humanized insulin gene. *Transgenic Res.* 19, 2, pp. (305-306)

Hrytsenko O, Pohajdak B, Xu B-Y, Morrison CM, van Tol B, & Wright JR Jr. (2010). Cloning and molecular characterization of the Glucose Transporter 1 in tilapia (Oreochromis niloticus). *Gen. Comp. Endocrinol.* 165, 2, pp. (293-303)

Hrytsenko O, Rayat G, Xu B-Y, Pohajdak B, Krause R, Rajotte RV, & Wright JR Jr. (2011). Lifelong stable human insulin expression in transgenic tilapia expressing a humanized tilapia insulin gene. *Transgenic Res.* – in press

Hrytsenko O, Wright JR Jr, Morrison CM, & Pohajdak B. (2007). Insulin expression in the brain and pituitary cells of tilapia (Oreochromis niloticus). *Brain Res.* 1135, 1, pp. (31-40)

Hrytsenko O, Wright JR Jr, & Pohajdak B. (2008). Regulation of insulin gene expression and insulin production in Nile tilapia (Oreochromis niloticus). *Gen. Comp. Endocrinol.* 155, 2, pp. (328-340)

Joy P. (2001). Cloning, sequencing, and expression of the tilapia glucokinase. MSc Thesis, Dalhousie University, Halifax, Nova Scotia, Canada

Leventhal JR, Sun JD, Zhang J, Galili U, Chong A, Baker M, Kaufman D, & Wright JR Jr. (2004). Evidence that tilapia islets do not express α(1,3) Gal: Implications for islet xenotransplantation. *Xenotransplantation* 11, pp. (276-283)

Lomedico PT, Rosenthal N, Kolodner R, Efstratiadis A, & Gilbert W. (1980). The structure of rat preproinsulin genes. *Ann. N.Y. Acad. Sci.* 343, pp. (425-432)

Mansour M, Wright JR Jr, & Pohajdak B. (1998). Cloning, sequencing and characterization of the tilapia insulin gene. *Comp. Biochem. Physiol.* 121B, pp. (291-297)

Morrison CM, Miyake T, & Wright JR Jr. (2001). Development of embryo and early larva of *Oreochromis niloticus* (Pisces: Cichlidae). *J. Morphol.* 247, pp. (172-195)

Morrison CM, Pohajdak B, Tam J, & Wright JR Jr. (2004). Development of the islets, exocrine pancreas and related ducts in the Nile tilapia, Oreochromis niloticus (Pisces: Cichlidae). *J. Morphol.* 261, pp. (377-389)

Morrison CM, Pohajdak B, & Wright JR Jr. (2003a). Structure and enzymatic removal of the chorion of embryos of the Nile tilapia *Oreochromis niloticus*. *J. Fish Biol.* 63, pp (1439-1453)

Morrison CM, Yang H, Al-Jazaeri A, Tam J, Plisetskaya E, & Wright JR Jr. (2003b). Xenogeneic milieu markedly remodels endocrine cell populations after transplantation of fish islets into streptozotocin-diabetic nude mice. *Xenotransplantation* 10, pp. (60-65)

Morsiani E, Lebow LT, Rozga J, & Demetriou AA. (1995). Teleost fish islets: a potential source of endocrine tissue for the treatment of diabetes. *J. Surg. Res.* 58, pp. (583-591)

Nguyen T, Wright JR Jr, Nielsen PF, & Conlon JM. (1995). Characterization of the pancreatic hormones from the Brockmann body of the tilapia - implications to islet xenograft studies. *Comp. Biochem. Physiol.* 111C, pp. (33-44)

O'Hali W, Yang H, Pohajdak B, LaPrairie A, Gross M, & Wright JR Jr. (1997). Cryopreservation of fish islets: the effect on function and islet xenograft survival. *Transplant. Proc.* 29, pp. (1990-1991)

Pohajdak B, Mansour M, Hrytsenko O, Conlon JM, Dymond C, & Wright JR Jr. (2004). Production of transgenic tilapia with Brockmann bodies secreting [desThrB30] human insulin. *Transgenic Res.* 13, 4, pp. (313-323)

Snel L & Damgaard U. (1988). Proinsulin heterogeneity in pigs. *Horm. Metab. Res.* 20, pp. (476-480)

Taylor JS, Braasch I, Frickey T, Meyer A, & Van de Peer Y. (2003). Genome duplication, a trait shared by 22000 species of ray-finned fish. *Genome Res.* 13, pp. (382-390)

Vaithilingam V & Tuch BE. (2011). Islet transplantation and encapsulation: an update on recent developments. *Rev Diabet Stud.* 8, 1, pp. (51-67)

Wolffenbuttel BH. (1993). The DCCT: "Metabolic control matters." Diabetes Control and Complications Trial. *Neth J Med.* 43, 5-6, pp. (241-245)

Wright JR Jr. (1992). Experimental transplantation using principal islets of teleost fish (Brockmann bodies). In: *Pancreatic Islet Cell Transplantation: 1892-1992 - One Century of Transplantation for Diabetes*, C Ricordi, RG Landes Co., pp. (336-351), Austin

Wright JR Jr. (1994). Procurement of fish islets (Brockmann bodies). In: *Pancreatic Islet Transplantation Series. Volume 1: Procurement of Pancreatic Islets*, RP Lanza and WL Chick, RG Landes Co., pp. (125-135), Austin

Wright JR Jr. (2002a). From ugly fish to conquer death: JJR Macleod's fish insulin research, 1922-24. *The Lancet* 359, pp. (1238-1242)

Wright JR Jr. (2002b). Almost famous: E. Clark Noble, the common thread in the discovery of insulin and vinblastine. *CMAJ* 167, pp. (1391-1396)

Wright JR Jr. (2006). Academic uses of GM fish technology: A call for a common sense approach to regulation. In: *Assessment of Environmental and Indirect Human Health Effects of Genetically Modified Aquatic Organisms*, RH Devlin, Canadian Technical Report of Fisheries and Aquatic Sciences 2581, Department of Fisheries & Oceans Canada, pp. (111-126), Ottawa

Wright JR Jr, Abraham C, Dickson BC, Yang H, & Morrison C. (1999). Streptozotocin dose response curve in tilapia, a glucose-responsive teleost fish. *Gen. Comp. Endocrinol.* 114, pp. (431-440)

Wright JR Jr, Bonen A, Conlon JM, & Pohajdak B. (2000). Glucose homeostasis in the teleost fish tilapia: insights from Brockmann body xenotransplantation studies. *American Zoologist* 40, pp. (234-245)

Wright JR Jr, Hrytsenko O, & Pohajdak B. (2012). Transgenic tilapia for islet xenotransplantation. In: *Aquaculture Biotechnology*, G. Fletcher and M. Rise, Blackwell Publications – in press

Wright JR Jr & Kearns H. (1995). Long-term culture, low temperature culture, and hyperoxic culture do not prolong fish-to-mouse islet xenograft survival. *Xenotransplantation* 2, pp. (19-25)

Wright JR Jr, Kearns H, Polvi S, MacLean H, & Yang H. (1994). Experimental xenotransplantation using principal islets of teleost fish (Brockmann bodies): Graft survival in selected strains of inbred mice. *Transplant. Proc.* 26, pp. (770)

Wright JR Jr, Kearns H, Yang H, Fraser RB, Colp P, & Rowden G. (1997). Immunophenotyping fish-to-mouse islet xenograft rejection: A time course study. *Ann. Transplant.* 2, 3, pp. (12-16)

Wright JR Jr, O'Hali W, Yang H, & Bonen A. (1998a). GLUT-4 deficiency and absolute peripheral resistance to insulin in the teleost fish tilapia. *Gen. Comp. Endocrinol.* 111, pp. (20-27)

Wright JR Jr & Pohajdak B. (issued 1/18/2000). Transgenic fish and a method of harvesting islet cells therefrom. US Patent No. 6,015,713

Wright JR Jr & Pohajdak B. (2001). Cell therapy for diabetes using piscine islet tissue. *Cell Transplant.*10, pp. (125-143)

Wright JR Jr & Pohajdak B. (issued 11/5/2002). Transgenic tilapia comprising a humanized insulin gene. U.S. Patent No. 6,476,290 B1

Wright JR Jr, Pohajdak B, Xu B-Y, & Leventhal JR. (2004). Piscine islet xenotransplantation. *ILAR J.* 45, pp. (314-323)

Wright JR Jr, Polvi S, & MacLean H. (1992). Experimental transplantation with principal islets of teleost fish (Brockmann bodies): Long-term function of tilapia islet tissue in diabetic nude mice. Diabetes 41, pp. (1528-1532)

Wright JR Jr, Snowden J, Hrytsenko O, Morrison CM, & Pohajdak B. (2008). Immunohistochemical staining for tilapia and human insulin demonstrates that a tilapia transgenic for humanized insulin is a mosaic. *Transgenic Res.* 17, 5, pp. (991-992)

Wright JR Jr & Yang H. (1997). Tilapia Brockmann bodies: An inexpensive, simple model for discordant islet xenotransplantation. *Ann. Transplant.* 2, 3, pp. (72-76)

Wright JR Jr, Yang H, & Dooley KC. (1998b). Tilapia -A source of hypoxia-resistant islets for encapsulation. *Cell Transplant.* 7, pp. (299-307)

Xu B-Y, Morrison CM, Yang H, & Wright JR Jr. (2004). Tilapia islets grafts are highly alloxan-resistant. *Gen. Comp. Endocrinol.* 137, pp. (132-140)

Xu B-Y, Yang H, Serreze DV, MacIntosh R, Yu W, & Wright JR Jr. (2005). Rapid destruction of encapsulated islet xenografts by NOD mice is CD4 dependent and facilitated by B-cells: Innate immunity and autoimmunity do not play significant roles. *Transplantation* 80, pp. (402-409)

Yang H, Al-Jazaeri A, & Wright JR Jr. (2002a). The immunoprotective effect of Sertoli cells co-encapsulated with islet xenografts is not dependent upon Fas-ligand expression. *Cell Transplant.* 11, pp. (799-801)

Yang H, Dickson B, O'Hali W, Kearns H, & Wright JR Jr. (1997a). Functional comparison of mouse, rat, and fish islet grafts transplanted into diabetic nude mice. *Gen. Comp. Endocrinol.* 106, pp. (384-388)

Yang H, McAlister VC, al-Jazaeri A, & Wright JR Jr. (2002b). Liposomal encapsulation significantly enhances the immunosuppressive effect of tacrolimus in a discordant islet xenotransplant model. *Transplantation* 73, pp. 710-713

Yang H, Morrison CM, Conlon JM, Laybolt K, & Wright JR Jr. (1999a). Immunocytochemical characterization of the pancreatic islet cells of the tilapia (*Oreochromis niloticus*). *Gen. Comp. Endocrinol.* 114, pp. (47-56)

Yang H, O'Hali W, Kearns H, & Wright JR Jr. (1997). Long-term function of fish islet xenografts in mice by alginate encapsulation. *Transplantation* 64, pp. (28-32)

Yang H & Wright JR Jr. (1995). A method for mass harvesting islets (Brockmann bodies) from teleost fish. *Cell Transplant.* 4, pp. (621-p628)

Yang H & Wright JR Jr. (1999). Co-encapsulation of Sertoli enriched testicular cell fractions further prolongs fish-to-mouse islet xenograft survival. *Transplantation.* 67, pp. (815-820)

Yang H & Wright JR Jr. (2002). Microencapsulation methods: Alginate (Ca^{+2}-induced gelation). In: *Methods of Tissue Engineering*, A Atala and R Lanza, Academic Press, pp. (787-801), New York

Yang H & Wright JR Jr. (2002b). Human beta cells are exceedingly resistant to streptozotocin *in vivo*. *Endocrinology* 143, pp. (2491-2495)

Yu W, Xu B-Y, & Wright JR Jr. (10/03/03). Directly vascularized pancreatic islet xenotransplantation: Is tilapia-to-nude mouse discordant? 7th International Xenotransplantation Congress, Glasgow, UK

Yu W & Wright JR Jr. (1999). Heterotopic cardiac xenotransplantation: fish-to-rat. *Xenotransplantation* 6, pp. (213-219)

Part 2

Genetic Engineering

3

Cloning of Homozygous α1,3-Galactosyltransferase Gene Knock-Out Pigs by Somatic Cell Nuclear Transfer

Hitomi Matsunari[1,2] et al.*

[1]*Laboratory of Developmental Engineering, Department of Life Sciences, School of Agriculture, Meiji University*

[2]*Meiji University International Institute for Bio-Resource Research*

Japan

1. Introduction

To overcome donor shortage in organ transplantation, xenotransplantation using organs of genetically modified pigs has been actively investigated (Ekser and Cooper, 2010). Thus far, the development of genetically modified pigs has mainly focused on overcoming the immune rejection of the xenograft. The creation of knock-out pigs lacking the xenoantigen α1,3-galactosyltransferase (GalT-KO) (Dai et al., 2002; Kolber-Simonds et al., 2004; Lai et al., 2002; Phelps et al., 2003) and transgenic pigs expressing complement regulatory factors (Fodor et al., 1994; Takahagi et al., 2005) has been successfully achieved.

We have produced genetically modified pigs by the heterozygous knock-out of α1,3-galactosyltransferase gene and the co-expression of two transgenes, human decay-accelerating factor (hDAF) and N-acetylglucosaminyltransferase III (GnT-III) (Takahagi et al., 2005). Natural breeding of the heterozygous GalT-KO pigs could produce live homozygous GalT-KO pigs (Fujimura et al., 2008a; Fujimura et al., 2008b; Takahagi et al., 2007) with the two transgenes. The three genetic modifications made to these pigs, namely, the GalT-KO plus expression of GnT-III and hDAF, should reduce rejection when their organs are used for discordant transplantation. More specifically, Galα1,3-Gal epitopes, which cause hyper-acute rejection, have been removed from the pig cells, thereby

*Masahito Watanabe[1,2], Kazuhiro Umeyama[1,2], Kazuaki Nakano[1], Yuka Ikezawa[1], Mayuko Kurome[3], Barbara Kessler[3], Eckhard Wolf[2,3], Shuji Miyagawa[4], Hiromitsu Nakauchi[5] and Hiroshi Nagashima[1,2]

[1]Laboratory of Developmental Engineering, Department of Life Sciences, School of Agriculture, Meiji University, Japan

[2]Meiji University International Institute for Bio-Resource Research, Japan

[3]Institute of Molecular Animal Breeding and Biotechnology, Gene Center, Ludwig-Maximilian University, Germany

[4]Division of Organ Transplantation, Department of Surgery, Osaka University Graduate School of Medicine, Japan

[5]Center of Stem Cell Biology and Regenerative Medicine, Institute of Medical Science, The University of Tokyo, Japan

reducing the antigenicity of the cells to human natural antibodies and suppressing the complement cascade reaction in the host. However, for the clinical application of xenotransplantation, it will be necessary to perform further genetic modifications in these pigs to overcome the various obstacles that exist in xenotransplantation (Ekser and Cooper, 2010; Klymiuk et al., 2010).

One strategy for achieving a more advanced genetic modification of the pigs is the use of somatic cell nuclear transfer (SCNT). This approach should make it possible to create pigs with multiple genetic modifications based on the existing GalT-KO/transgenic pig. Using the SCNT technology shown in Fig. 1, it should be feasible to introduce novel genetic modifications through sequential cloning. This approach might be used for removal of non-Gal antigens, controlling delayed xenograft rejection or cell-mediated immunity. In order to pursue such an approach, it is essential to know the reliability with which existing genetically modified pigs can be reproduced through somatic cell cloning technology. Here, we examined the feasibility of this strategy using three lines of GalT-KO pigs that had been created previously. We also describe the current efficiency of somatic cell cloning for generating genetically modified pigs for xenotransplantation research and discuss the prospects of applying this technology to achieve more sophisticated genetic modification of the pigs.

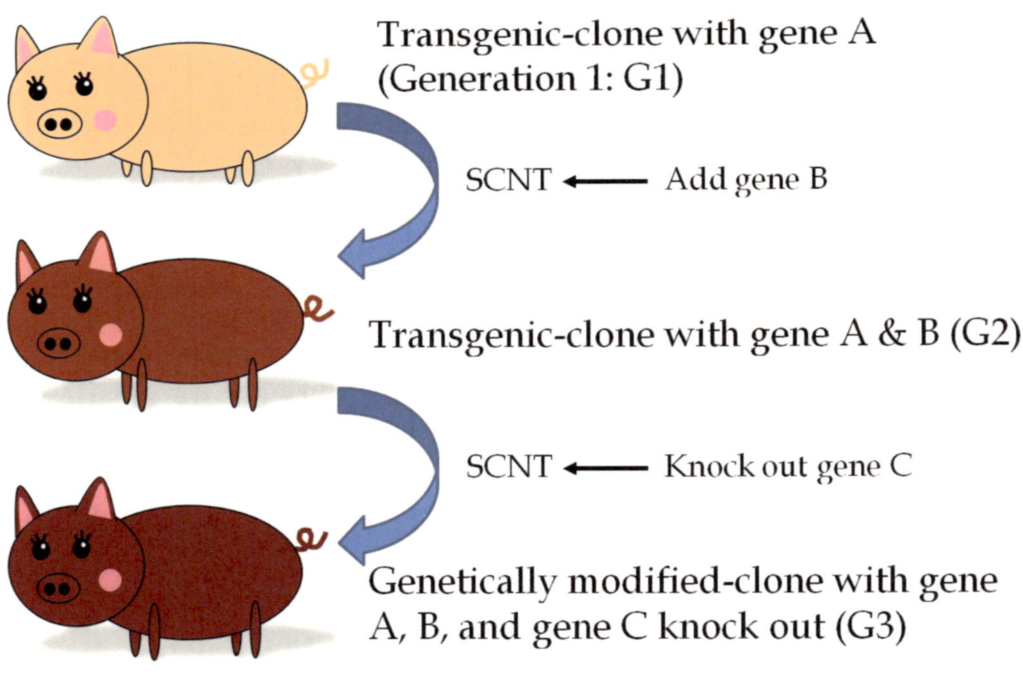

Fig. 1. Multiple genetic modifications of pigs using sequential somatic cell cloning

2. Reproducing GalT-KO pigs by cloning

In this study, we used somatic cell cloning to reproduce three types of GalT-KO pigs (DK3-1 male, DK3-2 female, DK3-9 female). These three types of pigs are all homozygous for the GalT-KO and were produced by intercrossing siblings derived from a mating of a heterozygous GalT-KO+hDAF+GnT-III pig to a wild-type pig (Table 1). DK3-1 and DK3-2 express two transgenes, namely, hDAF and GnT-III (Takahagi et al., 2005). However, the integration patterns of the two transgenes (i.e., heterozygous or homozygous integration) were not examined. By contrast, DK3-9 is a homozygous GalT-KO pig with no integrated transgenes.

Pig code number	Gal-T KO*	Transgenes**	sex
DK3-1	homozygous	hDAF and GnT-III	male
DK3-2	homozygous	hDAF and GnT-III	female
DK3-9	homozygous	NIL	female

*α1,3-galactosyltransferase gene knock out
** hDAF: decay-accelerating factor ; GnT-III: N-acetylglucosaminyltransferase III

Table 1. Original Gal-T KO pigs cloned by somatic cell nuclear transfer

3. Somatic cell cloning technology for reproduction of GalT-KO pigs

3.1 Nuclear donor cells for somatic cell cloning: Preparation of preadipocytes and cell cycle synchronization

Various types of primary cultured cells, such as fetal fibroblast cells, salivary gland progenitor cells and mesenchymal stem cells, have been used as the nuclear donor for somatic cell cloning (Faast et al., 2006; Kurome et al., 2008b; Matsunari et al., 2008b). For the cloning of GalT-KO pigs in this study, we used preadipocytes (Tomii et al., 2005; Tomii et al., 2009), which have consistently produced good results in somatic cell cloning in our laboratory.

Primary cultures of preadipocytes were established as reported previously (Tomii et al., 2005; Tomii et al., 2009) from the subcutaneous fat tissue of three homozygous Gal T-KO pigs at 6 months of age (Fig.2a, b). Subcutaneous fat tissue was collected by abdominal incision under general anesthesia and then washed with Dulbecco's phosphate-buffered saline (PBS; Nissui Pharmaceutical, Tokyo, Japan) supplemented with 75 μg/ml penicillin G and 50 μg/ml streptomycin. Connective tissue surrounding the fat was removed using sterile scissors (Fig. 2b). Small pieces of fat tissue were then excised and incubated in Dulbecco's Modified Eagle Medium (DMEM) with 2% (w/v) bovine serum albumin (BSA, Fraction V) and 0.1% (w/v) collagenase (Wako Pure Chemical, Osaka, Japan) for 1 h at 37°C (Fig. 2c). Dissociated cells were collected by filtration through 100-μm nylon mesh (Falcon 352360, Becton Dickinson, Franklin Lakes, NJ, USA). Following centrifugation at 150 *g* for 5 min, only mature adipocytes that remained in suspension near the surface of the supernatant were collected (Fig. 2d), and these adipocytes were washed several times. The mature adipocytes (1×10^5) were then incubated in a T12.5 cell culture flask (growth area, 12.5 cm^2; Falcon 353018, Becton Dickinson) filled to the brim with DMEM containing 20% (v/v) fetal bovine serum (FBS; JRH Biosciences, Lenexa, KS, USA) and tightly capped. The flask was inverted and incubated in a humidified atmosphere of 5% CO_2 in air at 37°C to encourage the adipocytes to attach to the inner ceiling of the flask (Fig. 2e). Following incubation for 7 days, morphological transition to a fibroblast-like shape, accompanied by a gradual decrease in the amount of cytoplasmic lipid droplets, was confirmed in cells attached to the flask's inner ceiling surface. Following confirmation of firm cell attachment, the flask was again inverted, and routine culture methods for adherent cells were implemented (Fig. 2f). The medium was changed every three days, and after two passages, preadipocytes were resuspended in fresh media supplemented with 10% (v/v) dimethyl sulfoxide (CELLBANKER® 1, Nippon Zenyaku Kogyo Co., Ltd., Fukushima, Japan) and were then frozen in liquid nitrogen.

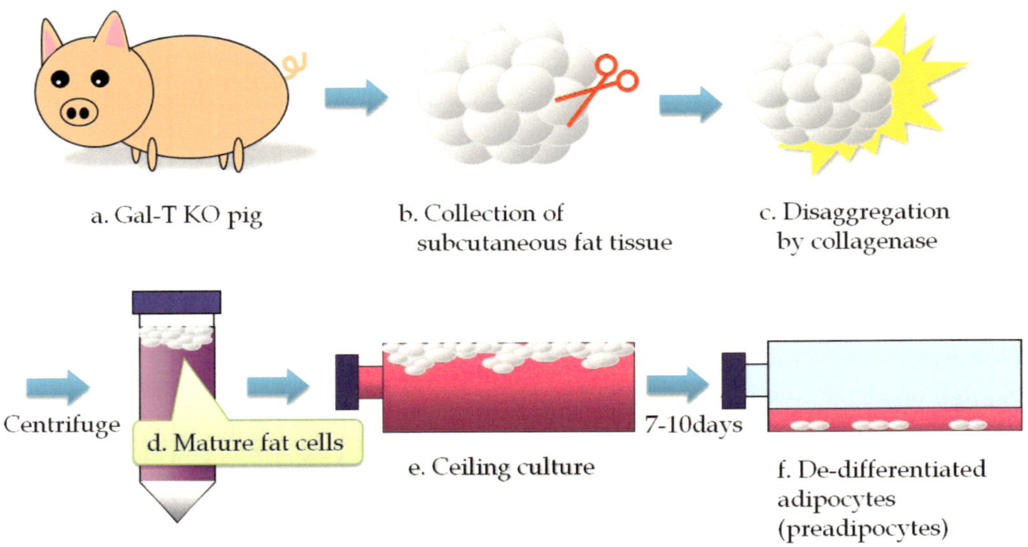

Fig. 2. Preparation of nuclear donor cells for somatic cell cloning from a GalT-KO pig: establishment of preadipocytes

After thawing by routine procedures preadipocytes were used as nuclear donors following cell cycle synchronization by serum starvation according to the method described previously (Tomii et al., 2005; Tomii et al., 2009); that is, preadipocytes were cultured in DMEM supplemented with 20% FBS to sub-confluence followed by culture for 2 days in DMEM with 0.5% FBS.

The ability of the obtained preadipocytes to re-differentiate into mature adipocytes was confirmed by the induction of differentiation *in vitro* (Tomii et al., 2005; Yagi et al., 2004). Sub-confluent preadipocytes were cultured for 4 days in DMEM supplemented with 20% (v/v) FBS, 0.5 mM 3-isobutyl-1-methylxanthine, 5 µg/mL insulin and 0.25 µM dexamethasone to induce adipogenic differentiation. After replacing the medium with DMEM containing 20% FBS, the cells were further cultured for 6 days. To examine the lipid droplet accumulation, cells cultured for 10days after differentiation induction were fixed in 10% (v/v) formalin and stained with Oil Red O for 20min.

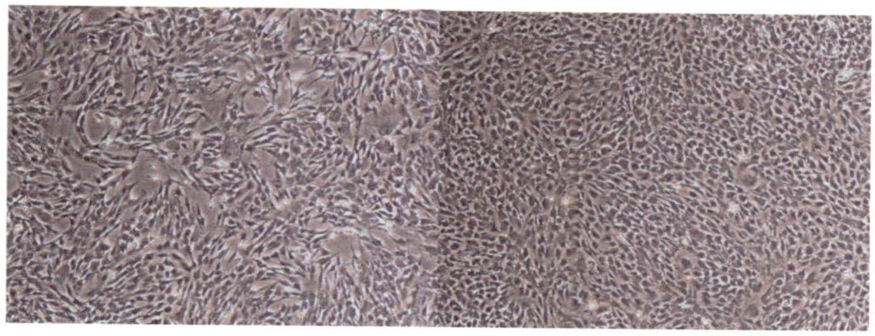

(a) day-0 (b) day-1

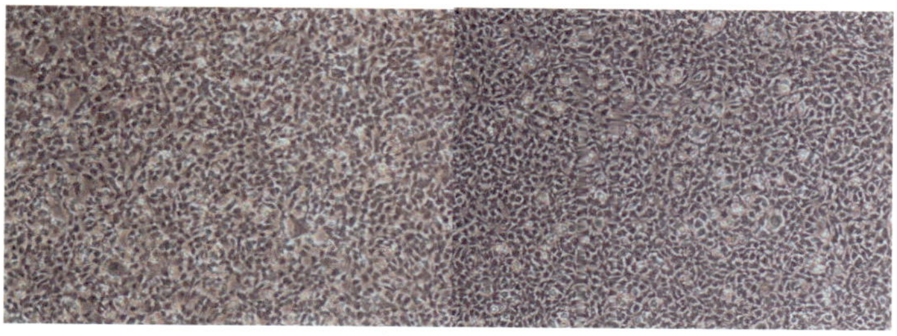

(c) day-3 (d) day-4

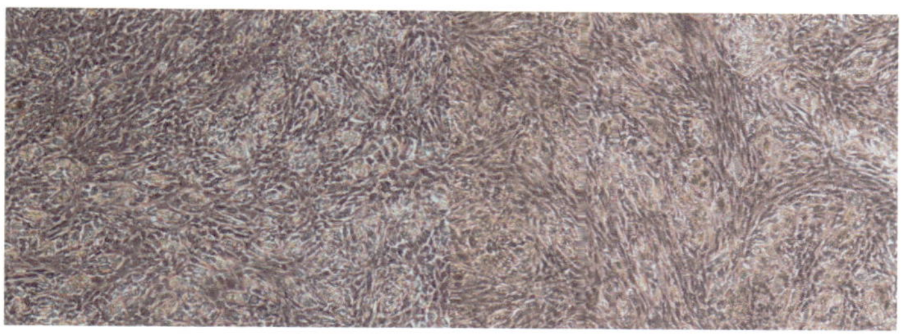

(e) day-5 (f) day-7

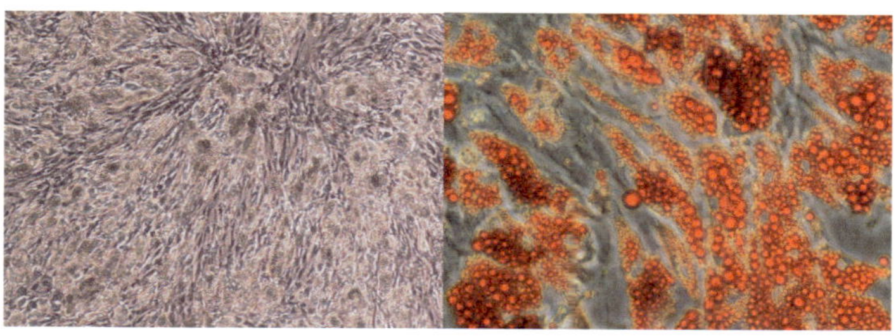

(g) day-10 (h) Oil Red O stained

Fig. 3. Re-differentiation of preadipocytes established from the GalT-KO pig (DK3-2)

Preadipocytes in sub-confluence before the induction of re-differentiation (a) and 1 to 10 days (b-g) after re-differentiation induction (x40). Re-differentiated cells on day 10 after fixation and staining (x200).

3.2 Karyotyping of nuclear donor cells

It is essential that the nuclei of the donor cells have a normal chromosomal constitution when creating somatic cell cloned animals. An examination of the cells showed that the normal chromosome number was present in 74% to 88% of the cells of the primary culture cell lines used in this study (Table 2, Fig. 4).

	DK3-1	DK3-2	DK3-9
Proportion of cells with normal chromosome number (2n=38)	74% (37/50)*	86% (43/50)*	88% (44/50)*

*Number of metaphase chromosome plates examined

Table 2. Chromosome composition of the nuclear donor cells used for somatic cell cloning of the Gal-T KO pigs

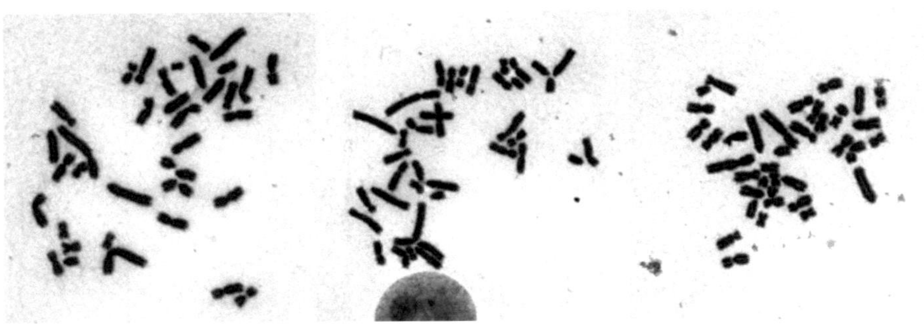

(a) DK3-1 (b) DK3-2 (c) DK3-9

Fig. 4. Normal chromosome numbers of the GalT-KO cells used for somatic cell cloning

3.3 Preparation of recipient oocytes for somatic cell cloning

Ovaries were recovered from gilts at a local slaughterhouse and transported to the laboratory in PBS containing 0.1% (w/v) polyvinyl alcohol (PVA), 75 μg/ml penicillin G, and 50 μg/ml streptomycin. Follicular fluid and cumulus-oocyte complexes (COCs) were aspirated from the follicles (diameter, 3 to 6 mm) using a 20-gauge needle attached to a 10-ml disposable syringe. COCs with several layers of compact cumulus cells were selected and cultured in NCSU23 medium (Petters and Wells, 1993) supplemented with 0.6 mM cysteine, 10 ng/ml EGF, 10 IU/ml eCG (ASKA Pharmaceutical, Tokyo, Japan) and hCG (ASKA Pharmaceutical), and 10% (v/v) porcine follicular fluid. Oocytes were cultured for 22 h with eCG and hCG in a humidified atmosphere of 5% CO_2 in air at 38.5°C and then for 18 to 20 h without these hormones in an atmosphere of 5% CO_2, 5% O_2, and 90% N_2 at 38.5°C.

3.4 Somatic Cell Nuclear Transfer (SCNT)

Nuclear transfer of preadipocytes was performed as described previously (Tomii et al., 2005; Tomii et al., 2009). *In vitro*-matured oocytes with expanded cumulus cells were treated with 1 mg/ml hyaluronidase and denuded of cumulus cells by pipetting. Enucleation was performed using a chemically assisted method developed by Yin et al. (Yin et al., 2002). Following culture in NCSU23 medium supplemented with 0.1 μg/ml demecolcine, 0.05 M sucrose (Nacalai Tesque, Kyoto, Japan), and 4 mg/ml BSA for 0.5 to 1 h, mature oocytes that had the first polar body were enucleated by aspirating the polar body and adjacent cytoplasm using a beveled pipette (diameter, 30 μm) in 10 mM HEPES-buffered Tyrode lactose medium containing 0.3% (w/v) polyvinylpyrrolidone (PVP), 0.1 μg/ml demecolcine, 5 μg/ml cytochalasin B (CB), and 10% FBS (Fig. 5a). When a protrusion was observed on the surface of an oocyte, it was also removed with the polar body (Fig. 5b). Enucleation was confirmed by staining the cytoplasts with 5 μg/ml bisbenzimide (Hoechst 33342).

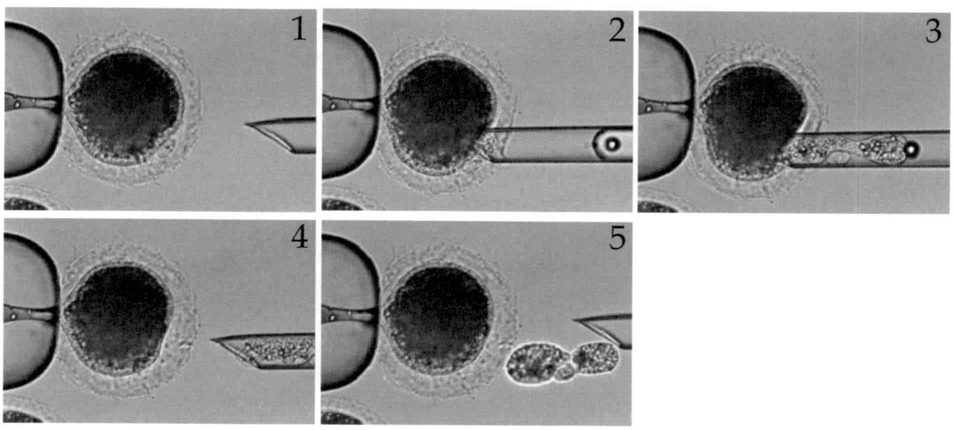

(a) Enucleation

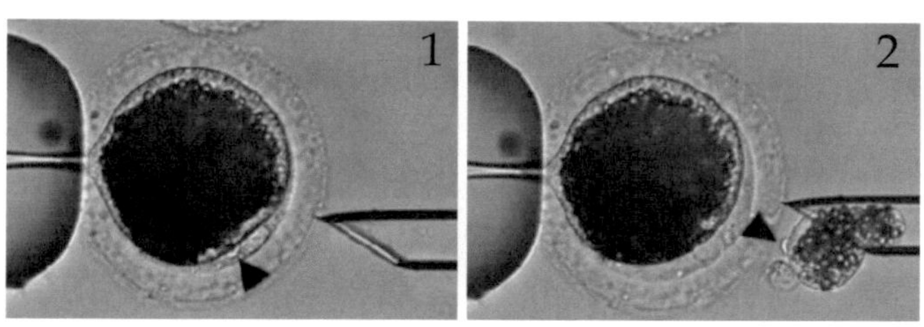

(b) Protrusion

Fig. 5. Enucleation of a porcine *in vitro*-matured oocyte: preparation of the recipient cytoplast for somatic cell cloning
(a) Removal of the first polar body and adjacent cytoplasm by aspirating with a beveled pipette (1-5)
(b) A protrusion (arrow head) visible on the surface of an oocyte was removed with the polar body (1-2)

Preadipocytes were used as nuclear donors following cell cycle synchronization by serum starvation for 2 days. A single donor cell was inserted into the perivitelline space of an enucleated oocyte (Fig. 6). Donor cell-oocyte complexes were placed in a solution of 280 mM mannitol (Nacalai Tesque) (pH 7.2) containing 0.15 mM $MgSO_4$, 0.01% (w/v) PVA, and 0.5 mM HEPES and were held between two electrode needles (Fig. 7). Membrane fusion was induced with a somatic hybridizer (SSH-1; Shimadzu, Kyoto, Japan) by applying a single direct current (DC) pulse (200 V/mm, 20 μsec) and a pre- and post-pulse alternating current (AC) field of 5 V, 1 MHz for 5 sec, respectively. The reconstructed embryos were cultured in NCSU23 medium supplemented with 4 mg/ml BSA for 1 to 1.5 h, followed by electrical activation. Reconstructed embryos were then washed twice in an activation solution containing 280 mM mannitol, 0.05 mM $CaCl_2$, 0.1 mM $MgSO_4$, and 0.01% (w/v) PVA and were aligned between two wire electrodes (1.0 mm apart) of a fusion chamber slide filled with the activation solution. A single DC pulse of 150 V/mm was applied for 100 μsec using an electrical pulsing machine (ET-3; Fujihira Industry, Tokyo, Japan). Activated oocytes were treated with 5 μg/ml CB for 3 h to suppress extrusion of the pseudo-second polar body.

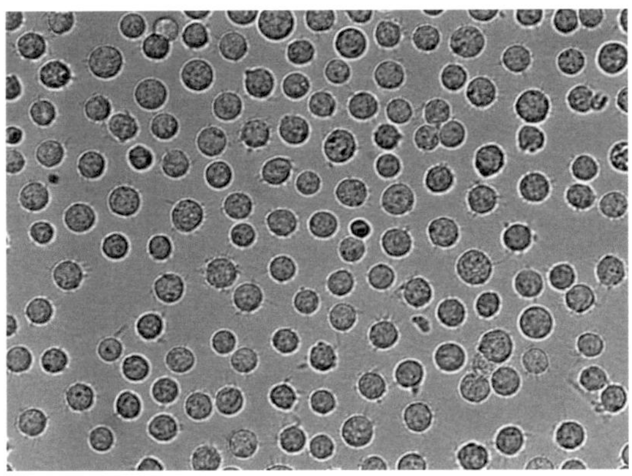

(a) Nuclear donor cells

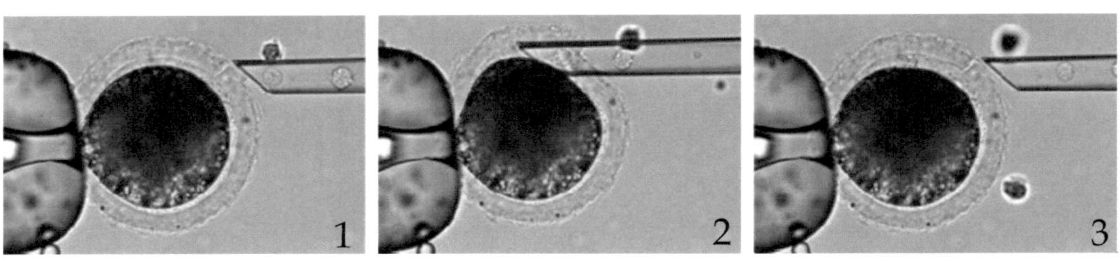

(b) Insertion of donor cell

Fig. 6. Insertion of nuclear donor cells into recipient cytoplast
(a) Nuclear donor cells derived from the homozygous GalT-KO pig (DK3-1)
(b) A single donor cell was inserted into the perivitelline space of an enucleated oocyte

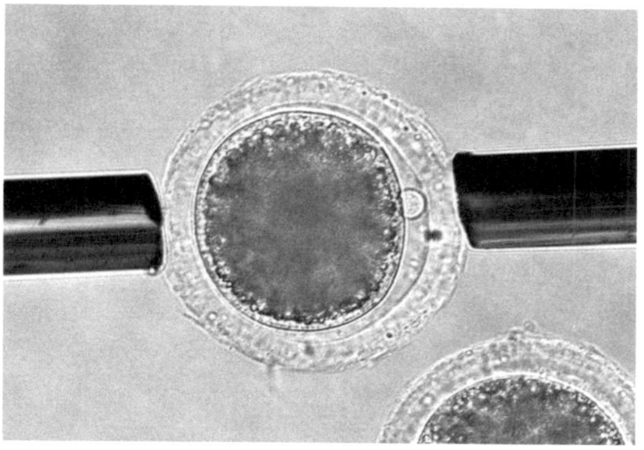

Fig. 7. Fusion of a nuclear donor cell and recipient cytoplast

An electric pulse was applied to a cell-oocyte complex using two electrodes (the chopstick method).

3.5 Culture of SCNT embryos

In vitro culture of SCNT embryos was performed in 20-μl droplets of PZM-5 (Functional Peptide Inc., Yamagata, Japan). The dish was maintained under a humidified atmosphere of 5% CO_2, 5% O_2, and 90% N_2 at 38.5°C. Beyond the morula stage, embryos were cultured in PZM-5 supplemented with 10% FBS. Cleavage and blastocyst formation of the reconstructed embryos were monitored during culture for 7 days. On Day 7, the number of cells in the blastocysts was counted after fixation and staining.

3.6 The effects of a histone deacetylase inhibitor on the development of SCNT embryos

Some of the SCNT embryos produced here were cultured in the presence of a histone deacetylase inhibitor (HDACi) Scriptaid, and their subsequent development was examined. The SCNT embryos, which had been undergone electrical activation and cytochalasin B treatment, were cultured in the presence of 500 nM Scriptaid in PZM5 for 15–20 hours and were then transferred to normal medium for further culture. The effects of HDACi were assessed by the rate of SCNT embryos that developed into blastocysts and the cell numbers in the blastocysts obtained.

3.7 Embryo transfer

Crossbred (Large White / Landrace × Duroc) prepubertal gilts weighing from 100 to 105 kg were used as recipients of the SCNT embryos. Gilts were treated with a single intramuscular injection of 1000 IU eCG (ASKA Pharmaceutical) to induce estrus. Ovulation was induced by an intramuscular injection of 1500 IU hCG (Kawasakimitaka Pharmaceutical, Kanagawa, Japan) given 68 h after the injection of eCG. Cloned embryos cultured for 1 or 2 days were surgically transferred into the oviducts of recipients approximately 51-54 h after hCG injection. Embryos cultured for 6 days were transferred at the blastocyst stage to the uterine horns of the recipients approximately 146 - 148 hr after hCG injection.

3.8 Analysis of cloned piglets

Homozygous GalT gene knock out in the cloned pigs was confirmed by PCR as described previously (Fujimura et al., 2008a; Fujimura et al., 2008b; Takahagi et al., 2005). Briefly, tail chips derived from the cloned pigs and a control non-transgenic pig were lysed overnight at 55°C in a lysis solution (10 mM Tris, pH 8.0, 1 mM EDTA, 100 mM NaCl, 0.5 % SDS, and 100 μg/mL Proteinase K). The lysates were extracted with phenol-chloroform followed by ethanol precipitation. The genomic DNA was resolved in TE buffer.

The primer sets used were the same as those described in previous reports (Fujimura et al., 2008a; Fujimura et al., 2008b; Takahagi et al., 2005). In the case of a targeted allele in which the GalT gene has been replaced with a marker gene (hygromycin-resistance gene), a DNA fragment of approximately 10 kb was amplified; however, in the case of the wild-type allele, a DNA fragment of approximately 7.6 kb was amplified. Amplification was performed on genomic DNA using the Expand Long Template PCR System (Roche; the forward primer was 5'-AGAGGTCGTGACCATAACCAGAT-3', and the reverse primer was 5'-AGCCCATCGTGCTGAACATCAAGTC-3'). After an initial denaturation step of 94°C for 2 min, PCR amplification was performed for 30 cycles of 94°C for 15 sec, 65°C for 30 sec and 68°C for 10 min with a 20-sec extension per cycle, and this was followed by incubation at 68 C for 7 min. Amplification products were analyzed by 1 % agarose gel electrophoresis.

4. *In vitro* development of cloned embryos derived from the GalT-KO pigs: An index for successful pig cloning

In vitro culture can provide an approximate estimate of the competence of SCNT embryos to develop into live cloned offspring. Since transcription from the embryonic genome starts around the 4-cell stage in porcine embryos, the early cleavage stages may be able to progress regardless of the existence of genomic aberrations. We found that the cleavage rate to the 2- to 8-cell stage in cloned embryos reconstructed from cells with numerical chromosome anomalies was similar to that of cloned embryos derived from normal cells (unpublished data). Although *in vitro* development into blastocysts does not guarantee the normalcy of the SCNT embryos, the ability to reach this developmental stage is nevertheless a reasonable indicator of whether cloned offspring can be obtained from the SCNT embryos. This raises the question of what rate of development of SCNT embryos into blastocysts is necessary to ensure that cloned pigs can be obtained. This question is difficult to answer as the culture conditions for embryos differ among laboratories. However, in our experience, when the developmental rate of cloned embryos produced using a given type of nuclear donor cell was over 30%, cloned pigs could almost always be obtained. With our porcine somatic cell cloning procedures, the *in vitro* developmental rate of the SCNT embryos into blastocysts exceeds 50%, and in such cases, the pregnancy rate of the recipients after transfer of the cloned embryo is almost 100%.

The *in vitro* development of the SCNT embryos is significantly improved by culture in the presence of a histone deacetylase inhibitor (HDACi), e.g., trichostatin A (TSA) and Scriptaid (Zhao et al., 2010). This improvement can be explained by the activation of transcription of genes involved in development, which results from histone hyperacetylation in the chromosomes of the cloned embryos. Table 3 summarizes the *in vitro* development of SCNT embryos created from GalT-KO cells. The blastocyst formation rate in the SCNT embryos derived from GalT-KO pig cells (DK3-1) was significantly improved (51.4 vs. 77.1%, P<0.05) by Scriptaid treatment. As shown in Fig. 8, the morphology of the cloned blastocysts treated with HDACi was better than that of untreated blastocysts, and the number of constituent cells was high.

Scriptaid treatment	No. of NT embryos cultured	Embryonic development (%)		Average cell number in blastocysts (mean ±SEM)
		Cleaved	Blastocysts	
+	35	27 (77.1)[a]	27 (77.1)[a]	70.9 ±6.5[a]
-	37	33 (89.2)[a]	19 (51.4)[b]	62.2 ±5.3[a]

[a, b]Values with different superscripts in the same column differ significantly

Table 3. *In vitro* development of porcine SCNT embryos treated with Scriptaid

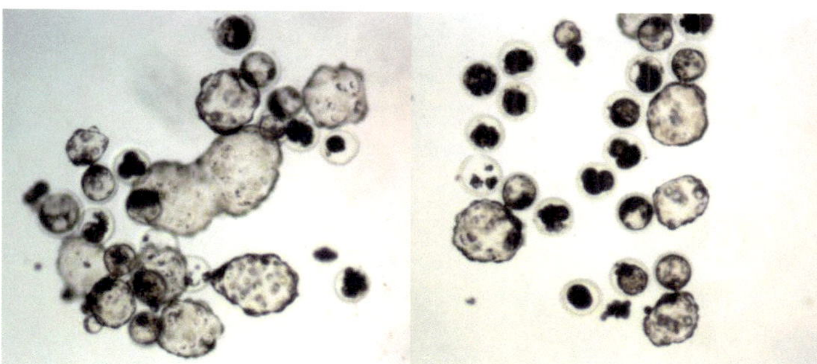

(a) Scriptaid(+) (b) Scriptaid(-)

Fig. 8. Morphology of cloned porcine blastocysts treated with Scriptaid

5. Creation of cloned pigs from GalT-KO cells

The results of transfer experiments with the cloned embryos are presented in Table 4. Transfer of the 547 cloned embryos reconstructed with the donor cells from DK3-1 into 6 recipients gave rise to 6 pregnancies (100%). Although 2 miscarried at 30 and 21 days of gestation, 2 recipients farrowed 10 piglets, including 2 stillborn piglets. From 2 other recipients, a total of 7 live full-term piglets were obtained by Caesarian section. The overall production efficiency of the cloned piglets was 3.1% from the recipients that farrowed or received a Caesarian section (17/547). Cloning efficiency of GalT-KO pigs in these experiments was comparable to that of non-KO pigs that we had reported previously (Kurome et al., 2006; Matsunari et al., 2008b).

As shown in fig., the DK3-1 cloned piglets were apparently healthy, though they were all sacrificed for analysis within 72 h. The average body weight and crown-rump length of the cloned piglets were 822.9 +/- 47.3 g and 24.7 +/- 0.5 cm, respectively (Table 5). The birth weights of the cloned pigs were much less than those of non-transgenic pigs with a common genetic back ground in our experimental farm (1.0 - 1 5 kg).

Origin of donor cell	Scriptaid treatment	SCNT embryos transferred	Recipients	Full term / Pregnant	Piglets or full-term fetuses* obtained (stillborn)**	Production efficiency of cloned offspring
DK3-1	-	547	6	4 / 6	17 (2)	17/547 (3.1%)
DK3-1	+	635	5	5 / 5	13 (5)	13/635 (2.0%)
DK3-2	-	176	2	2 / 2	2 (2)	2/176 (1.1%)
DK3-9	+	377	4	1 / 1	7 (0)	7/377 (1.9%)
DK3-9***	-	214	2	2 / 2	1(1)	1/214 (0.5%)

*Obtained by Caesarian section
**Within the piglets or full-term fetuses obtained
***Cloned embryos were produced from donor cells that were transported internationally

Table 4. The effects of Scriptaid treatment on the *in vivo* development of porcine SCNT embryos derived from Gal-T KO cells

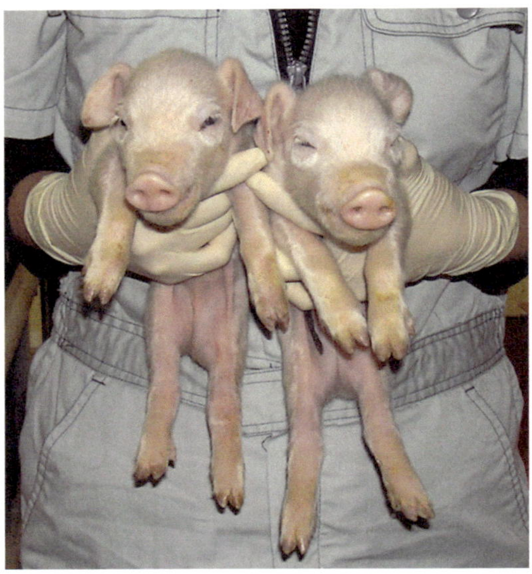

Fig. 9. Cloned offspring produced by SCNT of the homozygous GalT-KO pig cells co-expressing hDAF and GnT-III (DK3-1)

We also conducted an experiment in which cloned embryos, created using the cells from DK3-1, were treated with the HDACi Scriptaid and then transferred to recipients (Table 4). A total of 635 cloned embryos were transplanted into 5 recipients, all of which became pregnant (100%). By natural birth or full-term Caesarian section, 13 offspring were obtained from the recipients (5 were stillborn). The efficiency of producing offspring was 2.0% (13/635), indicating that HDACi treatment did not provide a marked improvement. However, it is notable that the six pregnant recipients did not have miscarriages in the experiment that used the HDACi treatment.

The body weight and length of the cloned piglets obtained from the 3 lines of GalT-KO cells are presented in Table 5.

DK3-1 Scriptaid (-)		DK3-1 Scriptaid (+)		DK3-2 Scriptaid (-)		DK3-9 Scriptaid (+)	
Weight (g)	Length (cm)	Weight (g)	Length (cm)	Weight (g)	Length (cm)	Weight (g)	Length (cm)
780	23	900	28	720*	23	1000	25
820	24	840*	25	480*	19	1000	26
820*	24	600*	23			1100	27
900	25	700*	25			900	25
1120	29	1500	27			700	23
580	23	1200	28			500	20
560	22	900	23			380	19
730	25	800	24				
1060*	27	900	25				
700	22	600	22.5				
700	23	600	24				
600	22	700*	26				
920	25	700	24				
1100	29						
900	25						
1120	29						
580	23						

*stillborn piglets

Groups	Average body weight (g) (mean± SEM)	Average body length (cm) (mean± SEM)
DK3-1 / Scriptaid (-)	822.9± 47.3	24.7± 0.6
DK3-1 / Scriptaid (+)	841.5± 72.0	25.0± 0.5
DK3-2 / Scriptaid (-)	600.0**	21**
DK3-9 / Scriptaid (+)	797.1± 104.2	23.6± 1.2

** SEM was not given due to limited sample numbers

Table 5. Body weight and length of the cloned piglets derived from the three types of the GalT-KO pigs

When 176 cloned embryos derived from DK3-2 were transferred into 2 recipients, both became pregnant, and 2 stillborn piglets were delivered (Table 4). The body weights and crown-rump lengths of these piglets were also much less than those of the normal piglets: 480 g compared with 720 g and 19 cm compared with 23 cm, respectively (Table 5). These stillborn piglets were delivered 2 days later than the expected date of farrowing. This delay may explain the weak DNA amplification signal obtained by PCR (Fig. 10).

Homozygous knock-out of the GalT gene was confirmed in all of the cloned pigs by PCR (Fujimura et al., 2008a; Fujimura et al., 2008b; Takahagi et al., 2005) (Fig. 10).

Transmission of the two transgenes, i.e., hDAF and GnT-III, was also confirmed in the cloned offspring. In the present study, we did not examine expression of these transgenes. However, faithful expression of transgenes in the cloned offspring produced by SCNT of a polytransgenic pig has been demonstrated in our previous studies (Fujimura et al., 2008a; Fujimura et al., 2008b; Takahagi et al., 2005). The influence of epigenetic modification on gene expression in cloned pigs needs to be investigated.

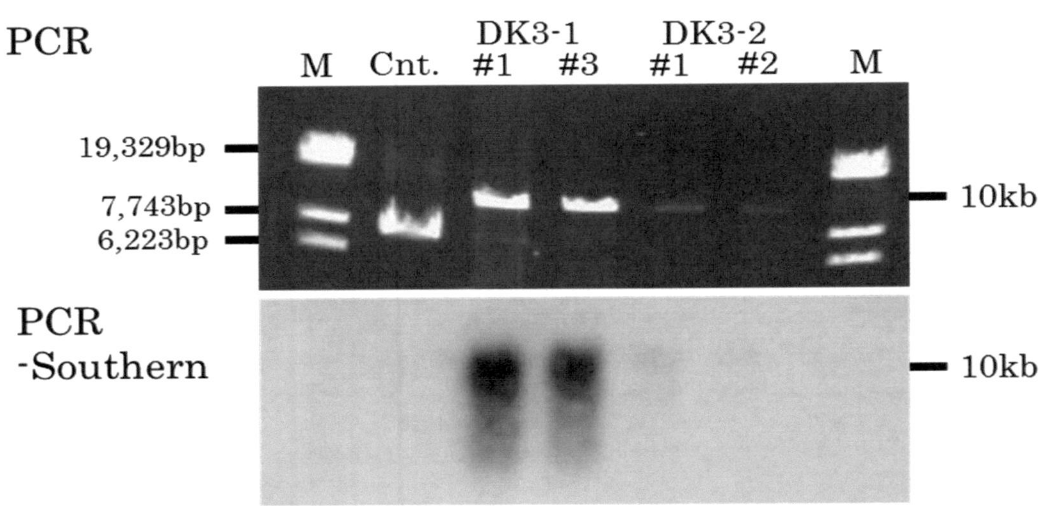

Fig. 10. PCR and PCR–Southern analysis of cloned pigs derived from homozygous GalT-KO pig somatic cells

Cloned pigs were produced from cells derived from DK3-9 (Table 4). DK3-9 is a GalT-KO homozygote and has no other genetic modification or transgene integration. The cloned embryos were treated with 500 nM Scriptaid for 15–20 hours. When 377 SCNT embryos were transplanted at the early cleavage stages (day 1 to 3), all 4 recipients became pregnant, and one sow farrowed seven live offspring. The average body weight and crown-rump length of the cloned piglets derived from the DK3-9 cells were 797.1+/- 104.2 g and 23.6 +/- 1.2 cm (Table 5). The other recipients had miscarriages. In the cloning experiments with DK3-9 cells, several miscarriages occurred, although the SCNT embryos had been treated with HDACi Scriptaid. This result is in contrast to the results of the cloning of DK3-1. It may be pertinent that the experiments with DK3-9 were performed during one of the hottest summers recorded in Japan, and this may have affected the recipients' pregnancies; further investigation will be necessary to identify the causes of the difference in experimental outcomes. Most of the cloned offspring with a normal range body weight were healthy and grew normally (Figs. 11, 12).

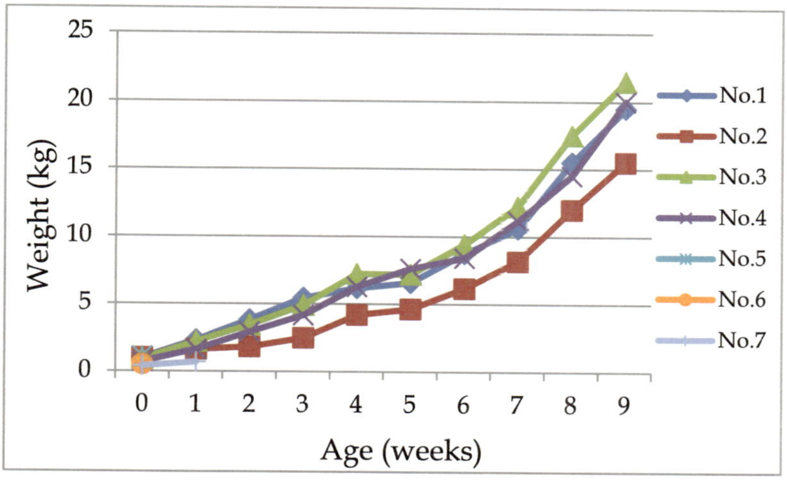

Fig. 11. Growth of the cloned pigs derived from the GalT-KO cells (DK3-9)

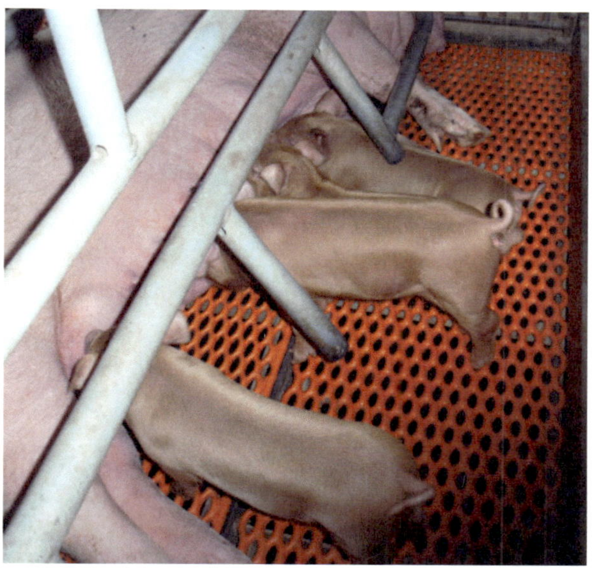

Fig. 12. Live offspring of a GalT-KO pig (DK3-9) produced by somatic cell cloning

The GalT-KO pig (DK3-9) cells that we created were transported by air from Japan to Germany and used to produce cloned pigs. As shown in Table 4, 214 cloned embryos were produced and transferred into 2 recipient sows. Both recipients became pregnant, and one cloned offspring was produced.

6. The prospect of the development of genetically modified pigs and the development of "rainbow pigs"

To bring xenotransplantation into clinical application, it is essential to overcome xenograft rejections, such as hyperacute rejection, delayed xenograft rejection, and cellular rejection

(Ekser and Cooper, 2010). Genetic modification of pigs by technologies based on SCNT would be the most promising approach to solve these issues. Furthermore, the advantage of SCNT is that additional genetic modification can be achieved based on the analysis of phenotypic expression of the resulting genetically modified pigs (Fig. 1). Genetically modified pigs so far developed as xenotransplantation donors including ours (Fujimura et al., 2008a; Fujimura et al., 2008b; Takahagi et al., 2005) will be further improved. With multiple gene modifications in pigs, the feasibility of serial somatic cell cloning (multi-generational cloning) would have important implications. In this regard, we have successfully produced the 4th generation of cloned pigs by serial cloning (Kurome et al., 2008a; Matsunari et al., 2008a). We have developed a process for multi-generational cloning of pigs, that is, a means of proceeding from the first clone generation (G1) to the second (G2) and then to the third generation (G3), and the efficiency of producing cloned pigs throughout this process was almost constant (Kurome et al., 2008a; Matsunari et al., 2008a). Notably, the cloned offspring did not show any shortening of their telomeres (Kurome et al., 2008a) and grew normally. Our results indicate that serial cloning is a feasible option for production of specifically designed pigs with multiple genetic modifications.

In this study, we investigated the feasibility of cloning the GalT-KO pigs by focusing on the introduction of multiple genetic modifications into pigs. The application of somatic cell cloning in xenotransplantation research is not limited to genetic modifications. Somatic cell cloning could also be used for reproducing large numbers of pigs with a preexisting genetic modification for use in organ transplantation experiments in primates and for other preclinical research (Kuwaki et al., 2005; Yamada et al., 2005). We have already started an organ transplantation experiment using the cloned GalT-KO pigs (unpublished). Additionally, as already discussed, while it is difficult to transport genetically modified pigs, it is a comparatively simple matter to transport cells from the pigs by air to overseas.

Development of genetically modified pigs has been attempted in several countries, including Australia, Britain, Germany, Japan, South Korea and the USA, with the aim of applying such animals in xenotransplantation. To realize their potential for clinical applications, it will be necessary to create pigs that incorporate all of the desired genetic modifications. We shall continue our pursuit of the ultimate goal of producing "rainbow" pigs—cloned pigs covering every possible genetic modification of medical interest.

7. Conclusion

In conclusion, the data presented in this chapter demonstrate that homozygous GalT-KO pigs can be efficiently reproduced by SCNT; hence, cloning technology is suggested to be a feasible option for proliferation of the genetically modified pigs. As part of the process of developing organ donors for xenotransplantation, somatic cell cloning provides an efficient and superior technology with high reliability and reproducibility for creating and reproducing pigs with multiple genetic modifications.

8. Acknowledgement

This study was supported by Promotion of Basic Research Activities for Innovative Biosciences (PROBRAIN), the JST, ERATO Nakauchi Stem Cell and Organ Regeneration

Project, Tokyo, Ministry of Health, Labour and Welfare, Tokyo, and Meiji University International Institute for Bio-Resource Research.

9. References

Dai, Y., et al. (2002). Targeted disruption of the alpha1,3-galactosyltransferase gene in cloned pigs. *Nature Biotechnology*, Vol.20, No.3, pp. 251-255.

Ekser, B. & Cooper, D. K. C. (2010). Overcoming the barriers to xenotransplantation: prospects for the future. *Expert Review of Clinical Immunology*, Vol.6, No.2, pp. 219-230.

Faast, R., et al. (2006). Use of adult mesenchymal stem cells isolated from bone marrow and blood for somatic cell nuclear transfer in pigs. *Cloning and Stem Cells*, Vol.8, No.3, pp. 166-173.

Fodor, W. L., et al. (1994). Expression of a functional human-complement inhibitor in a transgenic pig as a model for the prevention of xenogenic hyperacute organ rejection. *Proceedings of the National Academy of Sciences of the United States of America*, Vol.91, No.23, pp. 11153-11157.

Fujimura, T., et al. (2008a). Effects of recloning on the efficiency of production of a1,3-galactosyltransferase-knockout pigs. *The Journal of Reproduction and Development*, Vol.54, No.1, pp. 58-62.

Fujimura, T., et al. (2008b). Production of alpha 1,3-Galactosyltransferase gene-deficient pigs by somatic cell nuclear transfer: A novel selection method for gal alpha 1,3-Gal antigen-deficient cells. *Molecular Reproduction and Development*, Vol.75, No.9, pp. 1372-1378.

Klymiuk, N., et al. (2010). Genetic modification of pigs as organ donors for xenotransplantation. *Molecular Reproduction and Development*, Vol.77, No.3, pp.209-221.

Kolber-Simonds, D., et al. (2004). Production of alpha-1,3-galactosyltransferase null pigs by means of nuclear transfer with fibroblasts bearing loss of heterozygosity mutations. *Proceedings of the National Academy of Sciences of the United States of America*, Vol.101, No.19, pp. 7335-7340.

Kurome, M., et al. (2008a). Production efficiency and telomere length of the cloned pigs following serial somatic cell nuclear transfer. *The Journal of Reproduction and Development*, Vol.54, No.4, pp. 254-258.

Kurome, M., et al. (2008b). Production of cloned pigs from salivary gland-derived progenitor cells. *Cloning and Stem Cells*, Vol.2, No.3, pp. 277-286.

Kurome, M., et al. (2006). Production of transgenic-clone pigs by the combination of ICSI-mediated gene transfer with somatic cell nuclear transfer. *Transgenic Research*, Vol.15, No.2, pp. 229-240.

Kuwaki, K., et al. (2005). Heart transplantation in baboons using 1,3-galactosyl transferase gene-knockout pigs as donors: initial experience. *Nature Medicine*, Vol.11, No.1, pp. 29-31.

Lai, L., et al. (2002). Production of alpha-1,3-galactosyltransferase knockout pigs by nuclear transfer cloning. *Science*, Vol.295, No.5557, pp. 1089-1092.

Matsunari, H., et al. (2008a). Feasibility of serial somatic cell nuclear transfer in pigs. *Proceedings of Swine in Biomedical Research Conference*, pp. 37, San Diego, CA, USA, April 2-3, 2008.

Matsunari, H., et al. (2008b). Transgenic-cloned pigs systemically expressing red fluorescent protein, Kusabira-Orange. *Cloning and Stem Cells*, Vol.10, No.3, No. 313-323.

Petters, R. M. &Wells, K. D. (1993). Culture of pig embryos. *Journal of Reproduction and Fertility. Supplement*, Vol.48, pp. 61-73.

Phelps, C. J., et al. (2003). Production of alpha 1,3-galactosyltransferase-deficient pigs. *Science*, Vol.299, No.5605, pp. 411-414.

Takahagi, Y., et al. (2005). Production of alpha 1,3-galactosyltransferase gene knockout pigs expressing both human decay-accelerating factor and N-acetylglucosaminyltransferase III. *Molecular Reproduction and Development*, Vol.71, No.3, pp. 331-338.

Takahagi, Y., et al. (2007). Production of homozygous α1,3-galactosyltransferase gene knockout pigs co-expressing DAF and GnT-III. *Proceedings of the 10th Meeting of the Japanese Society for Xenotransplantation*, pp. 10, Tokyo, Japan, March 10, 2007.

Tomii, R., et al. (2005). Production of cloned pigs by nuclear transfer of preadipocytes established from adult mature adipocytes. *Cloning and Stem Cells*, Vol.7, No.4, pp. 279-288.

Tomii, R., et al. (2009). Production of cloned pigs by nuclear transfer of preadipocytes following cell cycle synchronization by differentiation induction. *Journal of Reproduction and Development*,Vol.55, No.2, pp.121-127.

Yagi, K., et al. (2004). A novel preadipocyte cell line established from mouse adult mature adipocytes. *Biochemical and Biophysical Research Communications*, Vol.321, No.4, pp. 967-974.

Yamada, K., et al. (2005). Marked prolongation of porcine renal xenograft survival in baboons through the use of alpha 1,3-galactosyltransferase gene-knockout donors and the cotransplantation of vascularized thymic tissue. *Nature Medicine*, Vol.11, No.1, pp. 32-34.

Yin, X. J., et al. (2002). Production of cloned pigs from adult somatic cells by chemically assisted removal of maternal chromosomes. *Biology of reproduction*, Vol.67, No.2, pp. 442-446.

Zhao, J., et al. (2010). Histone deacetylase inhibitors improve in vitro and in vivo developmental competence of somatic cell nuclear transger porcine embryos. *Cellular Reprogramming*, Vol.12, No.1, pp. 75-83.

4

Function Measurements of HLA-II Transgenic Pigs for Xenotransplantation

Hao-Chih Tai[1], Ching-Fu Tu[2,*], Tien-Shuh Yang[2], Jang-Ming Lee[1], San-Yuan Huang[2,3] and Bao-Tyan Wang[4]

[1]*Department of Surgery, National Taiwan University Hospital and College of Medicine*
[2]*Divisions of Biotechnology and Applied Biology, Animal Technology Institute Taiwan*
[3]*Department of Animal Science, National Chung Hsing University, Taichung*
[4]*Department of Genomic Medicine, Changhua Christian Hospital, Changhua*
Taiwan

1. Introduction

Using xenograft from transgenic (Tg) pigs is a promising approach to lessen the organ shortage for transplantation. Transgenesis such as CD55 or CD46, and CD59 as well as alpha 1, 3-galactosyl transferase gene knockouts shall avoid rejections. Indeed, grafts obtained either from hDAF (CD55) Tg pigs or from alpha 1, 3-galactosyl transferase gene knock-out pigs, all can overcome hyperacute rejection in xenotransplantation since porcine hearts could survive heterotopically in non-human primates more than 6 months (Kuwaki et al., 2005; Tai et al., 2007;). Obstacles are still remaining however, as early inflammation, acute humoral and acute cellular xeno-rejections and thrombotic microangiopathy are the following problems yet to tackle (Tai et al., 2007).

The early inflammation involves up-regulation of pro-inflammatory mediators in the graft and occurs before the T cell responses after engraftment. It is an innate response of NK cells to tissue injury and independent of the adaptive immune system. The major histocompatibility complex (MHC) molecules in human, including human leukocyte antigen (HLA) E, G, and class I molecules, in theory, can inhibit human NK cells xeno-rejection (Sasaki et al., 1999). This is proven by generating the HLA-E/human beta 2-microglobulin Tg pigs that can express transgenes consistently in peripheral blood mononuclear cells and on endothelial cells of organs, including heart and kidney, and these transgenes can provide partial protection against human NK rejections (Weiss et al., 2009).

In acute cellular rejection, T-cells cytotoxicity is responsible for the major cell-mediated rejections. In human allotransplantation, the donor-recipient match of HLA-II improves graft survivals, especially in kidney transplantation (Sheldon et al., 1999; McKenna et al., 2000). Yet, the roles of HLA-II to attenuate acute cell-mediated xeno-rejections remain uncertain. We have successfully generated HLA-DP, DQ and DR Tg pigs and showed that human-to-pig xenogenic cellular responses could be significantly depressed by expressing

*Corresponding Author

HLA-DP, -DQ or -DR exogenes on porcine cells (Tu et al., 2000a, 1999, 2000b, and 2001; Wang et al., 2004; Tu et al., 2003). The purpose of this review is an attempt to elucidate the functions of HLA-II in xenotransplantation.

2. The expression of DP or DQ exogenes in HLA-DP or DQ transgenic pigs reduced human-to-pig cellular responses

In allotransplantation, HLA-II matching could improve graft survivals, especially in kidney transplantation (Sheldon et al., 1999; McKenna et al., 2000), possibly due to better donor lymphocyte survival in recipients, so-called microchimerism (Starzl et al., 1992). However, the roles of HLA-II in porcine xenograft remain to be elucidated. In acute cell-mediated xeno-rejections, both direct and indirect pathways in human T-cell rejections are involving. The direct pathway, presumably the dominant one, engages in the early alloimmune response initiated by direct contact of host T-cells with allo-HLA molecules. Initially, human T cells recognize intact xeno-swine leukocyte antigens (SLA) on the surface of the antigen presenting cells (APC) or endothelial cells (EC) of transplanted pig organs. Then, human T cells identify xeno-SLA molecules bound xeno-peptide as being equivalent in shape to self-HLA bound foreign peptide and, hence, treat the xeno-tissue as foreign. In the proposed indirect pathway, human T cells recognize processed xeno-antigens presented as peptides by human APCs.

The roles of the HLA-II antigen in iso-, allo-, and xenotransplantation have also been studied in HLA-DQ and HLA-DP transgenic mice (Tsuji et al., 1994). The HLA-DP and DQ transgenic pigs were further produced through the technique of microinjection. Genomic DNA clones, including HLA-DP (including both A1 and B1 sequences) (Tu et al., 1999), and HLA-DQA1 and HLA-DQB1 (Tu et al., 2000) were transferred into pronucleus of porcine fresh fertilized eggs by microinjection. The successful integration of both HLA-DP and HLA-DQ transgenes were proven by polymerase chain reaction (PCR), Southern blot (Tu et al., 1999 and Tu et al., 2000, respectively), and FISH (Wang et al., 2004). The expression was also revealed by reverse transcriptase-PCR (RT-PCR) and by flow cytometry in HLA-DP (Tu et al., 1999 and 1998; Lee et al., 2000 and 2002) and HLA-DQ (Tu et al. 2003) transgenesis. To elucidate the function of HLA-DP and DQ antigens, the proliferation of human peripheral blood mononuclear cells (PBMC) to porcine xeno-antigen could be attenuated by primed or direct xenogenic mixed lymphocyte culture (MLC) tests.

The PBMC of the HLA-DPw0401 transgenic (Tg) pigs induced a stronger cellular reaction to HLA-DPw0401^{+}-primed lymphocyte test reagents than their non-transgenic (NTg) littermates. In direct xenogenic mixed lymphocyte culture (MLC) tests with responders from HLA-DPw0401^{+} humans, the PBMCs from the HLA-DPw0401 Tg pigs, as compared with those from the NTg littermates, induced low xenogenic cellular responses to human PBMCs (Figure 1). Furthermore, after 7 days of stimulation, the human responders (PBMC) without the HLA-DQw0601 allele displayed stimulating index (SI) of 1.37 ($\pm$ 0.53), 1.85 ($\pm$ 0.19), and 1.76 ($\pm$ 0.14) upon stimulation by PBMC from NTg littermates, wild pigs (WP), and third-party human (H) (HLADQ0601^{+}) respectively. Human PBMC responders bearing the HLA DQw0601 allele showed SI of 1.35 ($\pm$ 0.12), 1.42 ($\pm$ 0.09), and 1.10 ($\pm$ 0.16) upon stimulated by PBMC from NTg, WP, and H (HLADQ0601^{-}) controls, respectively ($p < 0.05$ for Tg versus WP, and Tg versus NTg). After 3 days of stimulation, the human PBMC responder without the human DQw0601 allele produced a higher level of INF-gamma when the stimulators came from the PBMC of WP, compared to Tg pigs (WP versus Tg: 55 ± 3.75 versus 24 ± 7.92 pg/mL). A similar trend was observed when the responders (PBMC) were obtained from the human DQw0601+ genotype (WP versus Tg: 153 ± 21.2 versus 69 ± 0 pg/mL). (Figure 2)

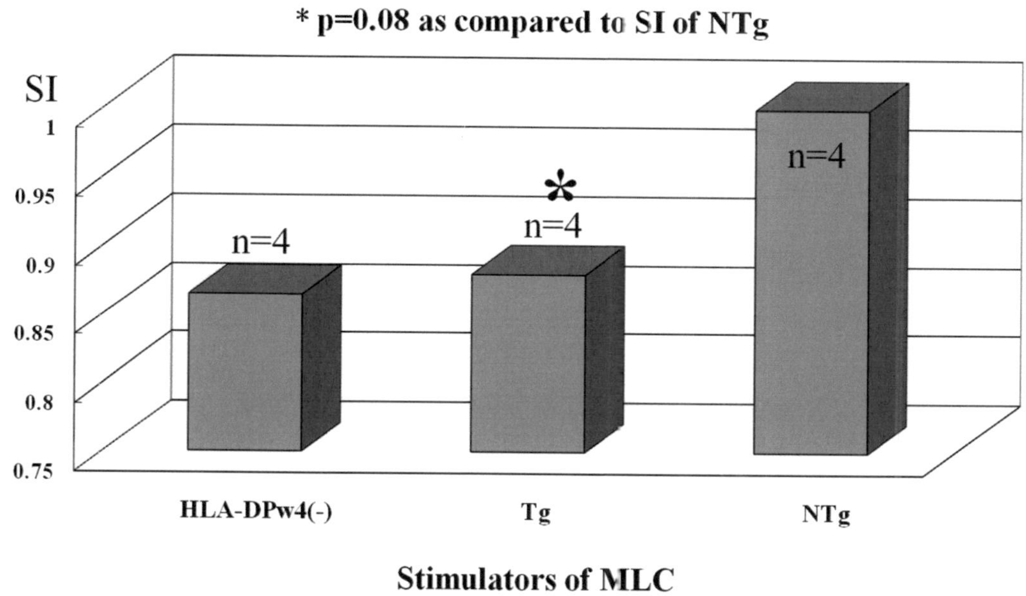

Fig. 1. Stimulating indexes (SI) of direct xenogenic mixed lymphocyte culture (MLC) test with responder of HLA-DPw4+ human lymphocytes. In direct xenogenic MLC tests with responders from HLA-DPw0401+ humans, the PBMCs from the HLA-DPw0401 transgenic (Tg) pigs, as compared with those from the non-transgenic (NTg) pigs, induced a lower degree of xenogenic cellular responses to human PBMCs. (n=4).

The cellular proliferation of human PBMC under stimulation by porcine PBMC was reduced in the presence of HLA-DQ molecules expressed on the porcine cells, as compared to that in the presence of the NTg littermate control. The human-to-porcine xenogenic Th1 response, as represented by the production of INF-gamma, was also attenuated by stimulation with HLA-DQ transgenic pig cells (Lee et al., 2003). These evidences were demonstrated in human PBMCs with or without the HLADQw0601 allele. The studies on the HLA-DPw0401 and DQw0601 transgenic pigs supported the concept that increasing the similarity of MHC class II determinants between HLA-II Tg pigs and human beings shall reduce the xenogenic cellular responses.

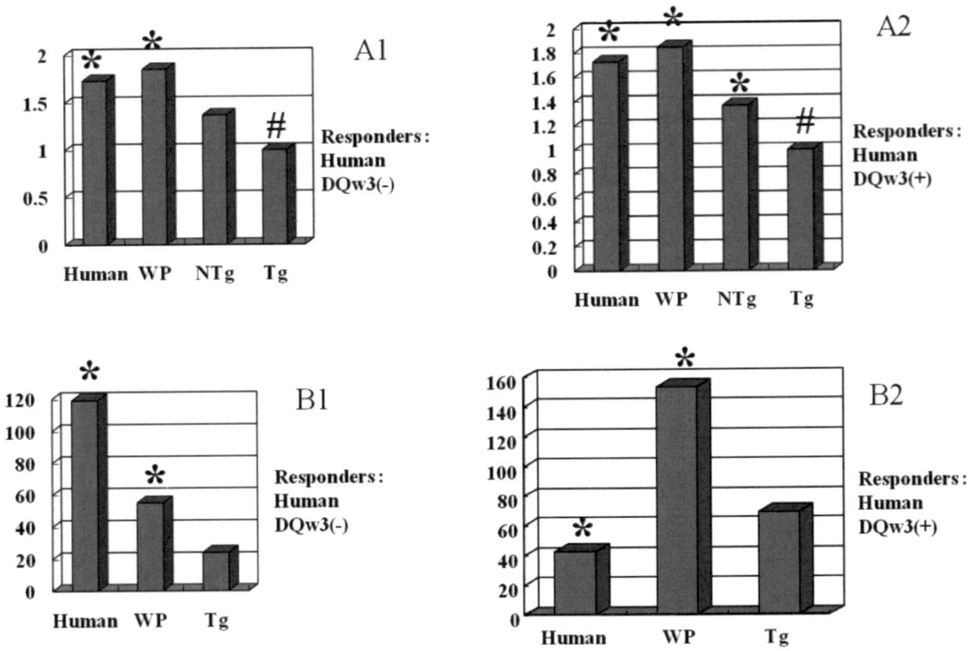

Fig. 2. Stimulating indices (SI) (A1 and A2) and TH1 response (INF γ production) (B1 and B2) of direct xenogenic mixed lymphocyte culture (MLC) tests with matched or mismatched responders of HLA DQw0601(+ or -) human PBMCs. A1 and A2: the cellular proliferation of human PBMC under stimulation by porcine PBMC could be reduced in the presence of HLA-DQ molecules expressed on the porcine cells, as compared to that in the presence of the NTg littermate control. B1 and B2: the human-to-porcine xenogenic Th1 response, as represented by the production of INF-gamma, was also attenuated by stimulation with HLA-DQ transgenic pig cells. Tg: HLA-DQ transgenic pig; NTg: non-transgenic littermate; WP: wild pigs; and each group n=3. * $p < 0.05$ as compared to Tg; # using the cpm of Tg as referent (SI=1).

3. The expression of DR exogenes in HLA-DR transgenic pigs enhanced cyclosporine effect

The integration of HLA-DR15$^+$ transgenes in transgenic pigs (Tu et al., 2001) was directly revealed by FISH which has localized both DRA1 and DRB1 transgenes on pig chromosome 13 near the centromere (unpublished data). The expression of transgenes has been confirmed by flow cytometry and the immunohistochemical stain. Results (unpublished data) have also shown that about 39.2% of porcine peripheral blood mononuclear cells and the endothelial cells on the blood vessel of transgenic pig successfully expressed HLA-DR antigens.

Proteomic approach (Huang et al., 2006) revealed that the HLA-DR15$^+$ transgenic pigs could express more proteins including triosephosphate isomerase, cyclophilin B (CyPB), proteaseme and RhoA than their non-transgenic littermates. It is of great interest to elucidate the association of HLA-DR with CyPB on transgenic pigs especially in xenotransplantation. Triosephosphate isomerase can stimulate lymphocyte proliferation

(Richter et al., 1993) and its minor structural change corresponds to substantially enhanced stimulation of a CD4+ tumor-infiltrating lymphocyte line (Sundberg et al., 2002). The proteasome is a multicatalytic complex of proteases involved in T-lymphocyte proliferation and activation and plays an important role in cell–cell interaction during T-lymphocyte activation (Kanaan et al., 2001). The GTP-binding protein RhoA is a member of the Ras GTPase superfamily and has been reported to be actively involved in the regulation of T-lymphocyte morphology and motility (Woodside et al., 2003). The Rho GTPases are molecular switches and are pivotal regulators of antigen-specific T-cell activation by antigen-presenting cells and immunological synapse formation (Deckert et al., 2005). The findings by Mzali et al. (Mzali et al., 2005) also suggested that Rho GTPases play crucial roles in T-lymphocyte functions and proliferation. These proteins are usually involved in T-cell activation or proliferation, except CyPB which belongs to a class of highly conserved proteins that accelerate the folding of proteins and being a cyclosporine A (CsA) binding protein (Schreiber, 1991). This protein is abundant in thymus cytoplasm and appears to be involved in the regulation of T-lymphocyte activation and proliferation (Harding et al., 1986), and inhibits the early T-cell activation (Liu et al., 1991) and prevents graft rejection (Schreiber and Crabtree, 1992). Furthermore, Denys et al. (1998) reported that plasma CyPB may enhance the immunosuppressive activity of CsA through a cell-mediated incorporation of CyPB–complexed CsA with in peripheral blood lymphocytes, and thus contributes to the acceptance and the good maintenance of organ transplantation. It is very interesting to elucidate the association of HLA-DR with CyPB on transgenic pigs especially in xenotransplantation.

By mixed lymphocyte culture, Tg and NTg pigs' lymphocytes (pLC, stimulator) were compared to stimulate activation of human lymphocytes (hLC; effectors) so that the survival of HLA-DR Tg pig endothelial cells (pETC) in contact with xenografting lymphocytosis could be further evaluated. The hLC from HLA-DR15+ or HLA-DR15- healthy adults with O- or B-type man or women, and from HLA-DR15+ Tg and NTg pLC were harvested from peripheral blood samples by Ficoll-Paque™ Plus and separated from hematopoietic cells by culturing in 35 mm dish for overnight. Porcine LC was inactivated by 10.0 μg/mL of mitomycin C for 30 min before mixed with hLC. These xeno-mixed LC reactions were cultivated in RPMI1640 medium adding 0, 0.1 and 1 μg/mL of CsA and for 48 hours. The proliferation of hLC was evaluated by MTS assay. Results (Figure 3) thus obtained were: without CsA, the pLC stimulated 1.2 ±2.0 ~ 47.0 ±4.0% of hLC proliferation; while after addition of 0.1 and 1 μg/mL CsA, the Tg vs. NTg pLC enhanced inhibition effects on hLC proliferation was 23.8 ±2.5 ~ 23.8 ±2.9% vs. 14.7 ±2.5 ~ 14.9 ±2.5%, and at 47.9 ±2.4 ~ 48.1 ±2.8% vs. 24.9 ±2.0 ~28.5 ±2.4%, respectively. Result showed that inactivation of hLC by CsA could be enhanced by HLA-DR transgenesis, suggesting that an ameliorated effect has occurred in acute xenograft rejection. The expression of CyPB in HLA-DR transgenic lymphocytes (intracellular) (Huang et al., 2006) could depress hLC activation. However, the improvement of survival rate of pETC (responder) varied highly in Tg pETC as compared to NTg pETC (data not shown). Although CyPB was expressed on endothelial cells (Carpentieret et al., 1999) and capable of enhancing T-cell adhesion to ETC extracellular matrix, then it could significantly attenuate by CsA (Allain et al., 2002). It is worth noting that HLA-DR transgenesis and the expression and secretion of CyPB on pETC will be firstly attached by activated hLC.

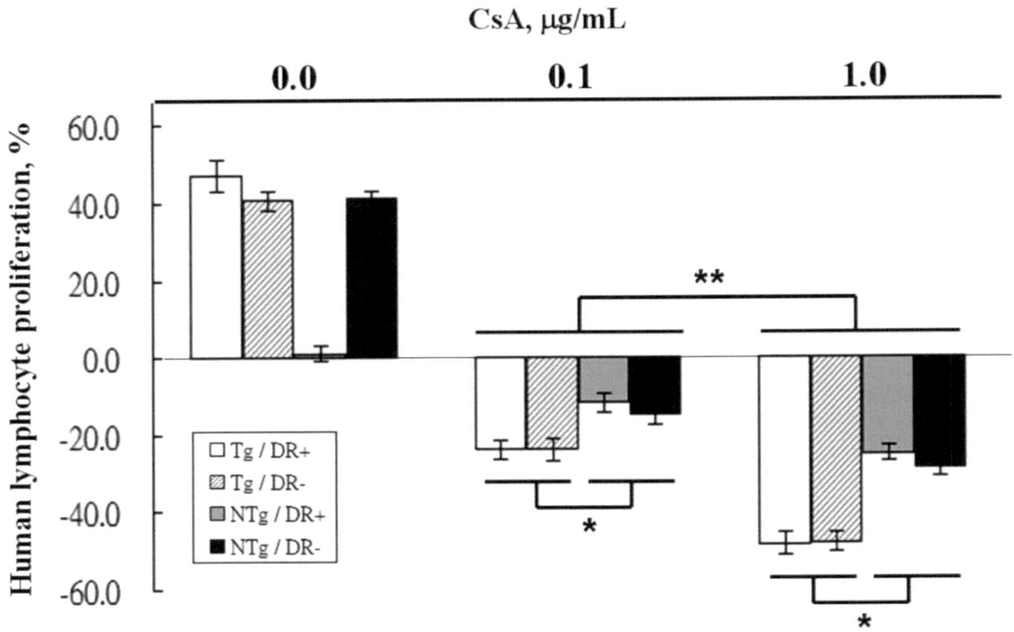

Fig. 3. Human lymphocytes mixed reaction with HLA-DR15+ transgenic (Tg) or non-Tg (NTg) lymphocytes. The surface antigens on human lymphocytes were with DR15+ or DR15-. There were 0, 0.1 and 1.0 μg/mL immuosuppressor, CsA, added into the medium of mixed lymphocytes culture tests to evaluate the synergic effects of transgenes. N= 3; * $p < 0.05$ and ** $p < 0.01$.

4. Long-term survival of HLA-DR pig skin in SCID mice after reconstitution with human PBMC and under short-term immunosuppression

To test the role of donor-recipient HLA-II-match in xenotransplantation, the HLA-DR15+ porcine skins were transplanted to SCID mice which were thereafter reconstituted with HLA-DR 15+ or DR15- hPBMC. The studies were conducted under no immunosuppression (no CsA was given to hPBMC-SCID mice), or under immunosuppression (CsA was given intra-peritoneally to hPBMC-SCID mice for 12 days) to reveal the effectiveness of the graft.

In studies of HLA-DR15+ porcine skin grafts to hPBMC-SCID mice under no immunosuppression (Tu et al., 2008), human CD4+ and CD8+ cells were detected from days 7 to 29 after hPBMC reconstitution in hPBMC-SCID mice. Both CD4+ and CD8+ cells of HLA-DR15- hPBMC-SCID mice were significantly higher at day 29 post-grafting, compared with that of HLA-DR15+ hPBMC-SCID mice. In HLA-DR15+ hPBMC-SCID mice, the HLA-DR15+ Tg pig skin grafts survived and integrated into mice, and illustrated histopathologically less cellular rejections which showed intact dermis with little lymphocytic infiltration. However, in HLA-DR15- hPBMC-SCID mice, the HLA-DR15+ transgenic pig skin grafts illustrated more cellular rejections which showed disrupted collagen, as well as mild to moderate lymphocytic infiltration. The results suggested that HLA-DR matching attenuated xenogenic cellular rejection.

In studies of HLA-DR15$^+$ porcine skin grafts to hPBMC-SCID mice under immunosuppression with CsA (Tai et al., 2008), human CD4$^+$ and CD8$^+$ cells were found in hPBMC-SCID mice after reconstitution. Tests of MLC showed more responses of HLA-DR15$^-$ hPBMC against HLA-DR15$^+$ porcine PBMC. HLA-DR15$^+$ porcine skin grafts survived more than 100 days in hPBMC-SCID mice which were reconstituted twice with HLA-DR15$^+$ or HLA-DR15$^-$ hPBMC. In the negative control group, HLA-DR15$^+$ porcine skins were rejected in all non-SCID (Balb/c) mice (data not shown), and the gross pictures showed disappeared porcine skin and growth of murine hair in non-SCID (Balb/c) mice. Histological pictures of transplanted HLA-DR15$^+$ porcine skin grafts showed survived porcine epithelium in remodeling murine dermis (with organized collagen), and little lymphocytes infiltration in murine dermis.

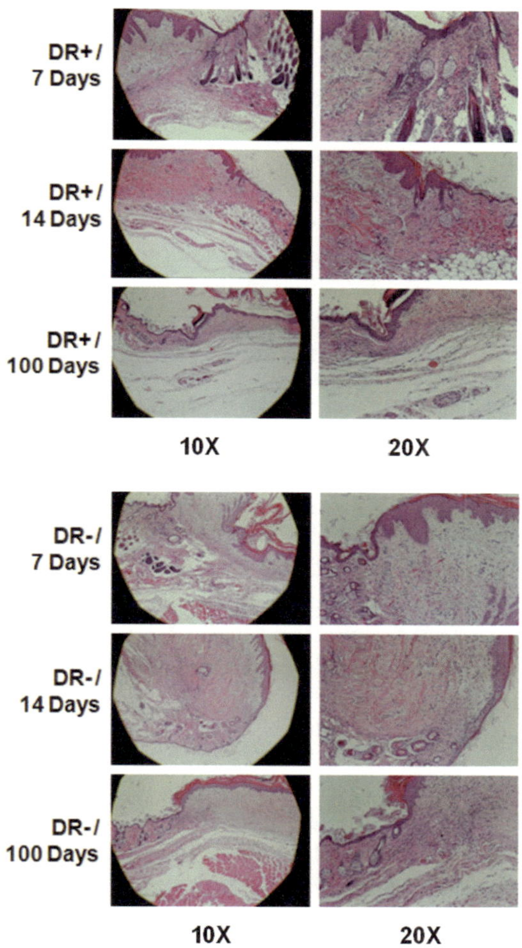

Fig. 4. Histological pictures (H&E staining) of transplanted HLA-DR15$^+$ pig skin showed survived porcine epithelium in remodeling murine dermis (with organized collagen), and little lymphocytes infiltration in murine dermis. (DR+: reconstitution with HLA-DR 15$^+$ hPBMC; DR-: reconstitution with HLA-DR 15$^-$ hPBMC.)

Although the results do not suggest that HLA-DR matching attenuated xenogenic cellular rejection, it showed that HLA-DR15$^+$ pig skin grafts could survive over a prolonged period in hPBMC-SCID under a short period of immunosuppression with CsA. The long-term survival of HLA-DR15$^+$ pig skin grafts in either HLA-DR15$^+$ or HLA-DR15$^-$ hPBMC-SCID mice might be due to poor engraftment or function of reconstituted T cells, under immunosuppression with CsA. Because of the gradually decreased number of reconstituted T cells and suppression effect of CsA, HLA-DR15$^+$ pig skin grafts were not rejected and therefore survived more than 100 days. In studies of T cell proliferation responses to porcine aortic endothelial cells (PAEC) either in the presence or absence of CsA, both allogeneic and xenogeneic T cell responses could be inhibited by in vitro (Fig. 3) or by therapeutic levels of CsA in vivo (Batten et al., 1999).

In the studies of Hagihara et al. (1996), in vitro MLC and in vivo skin grafting were conducted by using HLA-DP Tg mice (B6-DP mice). Xenogenic iso-(B6-DP to B6 mice) MLC showed positive but much less responses when compared to allo-MLC responses. Nevertheless, B6-DP skin grafts were rejected in a similar time period as allo-skin grafts. Further studies of in vitro cytotoxic lymphocyte responses and delayed-type hypersensitivity reactions indicated that xenogeneic HLA-DP antigens could act as significant transplantation antigens equivalent to alloantigens despite their less stimulative activity in vitro. Results also support the interpretation that DP antigens act like a minor histocompatibility antigen beyond the difference of species (Hagihara et al., 1996). In our studies, xenogenic HLA-DR15$^+$ antigens which act as minor histocompatibility antigens and swine leukocyte antigens (SLA) contributed simultaneously to exert acute cellular rejection of porcine skins in hPBMC-SCID mice.

During allogenic skin rejection, the destruction of critical dermal structures that determine the ultimate viability of the skin graft is highly antigen-specific and is almost certainly accomplished by cytotoxic T cells. Whereas destruction of non-critical epidermal structures of the skin allograft is antigen-nonspecific and can be accomplished by inflammatory cells or their secreted products. The MHC antigens are specific antigens for skin rejection. Matched MHC antigens of donors and recipients may improve survivals of allogenic skin graft. The in vivo skin-grafting in HLA-DR15$^+$ hPBMC-SCID mice, matched HLA-DR15$^+$ transgenic pig skin grafts displayed less cellular rejections.

5. Summary and conclusion

Our results from studies on the HLA-DPw0401 and HLA-DQw0601 Tg pig support the concept that increasing the similarity of MHC class II determinants between pig and human using an HLA-II Tg pig could reduce the xenogenic cellular response and attenuate human lymphocytic proliferation in xeno-mixed lymphocyte cultures and human-to-pig xenogenic cellular responses. In addition, proteomic approaches revealed that the HLA-DR15$^+$ transgenic pigs could express more proteins including triosephosphate isomerase, cyclophilin B (CyPB), proteaseme and RhoA than their non-transgenic littermates. These proteins are involved in T-cell activation or proliferation, except CyPB which belongs to a class of highly conserved proteins that accelerate the folding of proteins and being a cyclosporine A (CsA) binding protein. This protein is abundant in thymus cytoplasm and appears to engage in the regulation of T-lymphocyte activation and proliferation, and inhibits the early T-cell activation and prevents graft rejection. Furthermore, the plasma CyPB may enhance the immunosuppressive activity of CsA through a cell-mediated incorporation of CyPB–complexed CsA within peripheral blood lymphocytes, and thus contributes to the acceptance and the good maintenance of organ transplanted. By using in vitro mixed xeno-lymphocytes culture, the inactivation of hLC by CsA could be enhanced by HLA-DR transgenesis, suggesting that an ameliorated effect has occurred in acute xenograft rejection. Further studies using in vivo skin-grafting in HLA-DR15+ hPBMC-SCID mice, HLA-DR15+ Tg pig skin grafts displayed less cellular rejections due to additional histocompatibility factor, HLA-DR15+, especially at the administration of CsA.

6. Acknowledgements

The project was jointly initiated by professor Kimiyoshi Tsuji of Tokai University of Japan and late professor Chun-Jean Lee of National Taiwan University in 1994. Their inspirations and encouragements are very much appreciated. Financial supports by National Science Council, Executive Yuan, Taiwan, ROC, are gratefully acknowledged. Sincere thanks are also due to Mr. Takayuki Sato for his expertise in preparation of injection DNA and to Ms YH Chen, MS Liu, CP Wu, LL Ho, WT Lien, and WR Chang for their skillful assistances in generation of transgenic animals, in vitro study, and skin-graft animal trials. The suggestions on the data statistics by Dr. SF Guo are also appreciated.

7. References

[1] Allain F., C. Vanpouille, M. Carpentier, M.-C. Slomianny, S. Durieux, and G. Spik. Interaction with glycosaminoglycans is required for cyclophilin B to trigger integrin-mediated adhesion of peripheral blood T lymphocytes to extracellular matrix. PNAS, 2002 ; 99: 2714-2719.

[2] Batten P, McCormack AM, Page CS, Yacoub MH, Rose ML. Human T cell responses to human and porcine endothelial cells are highly sensitive to cyclosporin A and FK506 in vitro. Transplantation. 1999; 68: 1552-1560.

[3] Carpentier, M., Descamps, L., Allain, F., Denys, A., Durieux, S., Fenart, L., Kieda, C., Cecchelli, R. and Spik, G. Receptor-mediated transcytosis of cyclophilin B through the blood-brain barrier. J. Neurochem. 1999, 73: 260–270.

[4] Deckert M, Moon C, and Le Bras S. The Immunological Synapse and Rho GTPases. Curr. Top. Microbiol. Immunol. 2005, 291, 61–90.

[5] Denys A, Allain F, Masy E, Dessaint JP, Spik G. Enhancing the effect of secreted cyclophilin B on immunosuppressive activity of cyclosporine. Transplantation. 1998; 65: 1076-1084.

[6] Hagihara M, Shimura T, Takebe K, Munkhbat B, Sato T, Tsuchida F, Sato K, Tsuji K. Xenogeneic iso-skin graft and mixed lymphocyte reaction studies using HLA-DP transgenic mice. Transpl Immunol. 1996; 4: 220-226.

[7] Harding MW, Handschumacher RE, and Speicher DW. Isolation and amino acid sequence of cyclophilin. J Biol Chem. 1986; 261: 8547-8555.

[8] Huang SY, Chen YH, Teng SH, Chen IC, Ho LL, Tu CF. Protein expression of lymphocytes in HLA-DR transgenic pigs by a proteomic approach. Proteomics 2006; 6: 5815-5825.
[9] Kanaan N, Luo H, Wu J. Proteasome activity is required for T lymphocyte aggregation after mitogen activation. J Cell Biochem. 2001; 81: 347-356.
[10] Kuwaki K, Tseng YL, Dor FJMF, Shimizu A, Houser SL, Sanderson TM, Lancos CJ, Prabharasuth DD, Cheng J, Moran K, Hisashi Y, Mueller N, Yamada K, Greenstein JL, Hawley RJ, Patience C, Awwad M, Fishman JA, Robson SC, Schuurman HJ, Sachs DH, and Cooper DK. Heart transplantation in baboons using α1,3-galactosyltransferase gene-knockout pigs as donors: initial experience. Nat Med. 2005; 11: 29-31.
[11] Lee JM, Tu CF, Yang PW, Lee YC, Lee CJ. The effective antigen presentation of human MHC on the lymphocytes of HLA DPW0401 transgenic pigs: examination with xenogenic mixed lymphocyte culture and primed lymphocyte tests. Transplant Proc. 2000; 32: 2503-2504.
[12] Lee JM, Tu CF, Yang PW, Lee KH, Tsuji K, Tsai MK, Chen RJ, Hu CY, Hsieh RP, Tai HC, Chiang BL, Weng CN, Lee YC, Lee CJ. Reduction of human-to-pig cellular response by alteration of porcine MHC with human HLA DPW0401 exogenes. Transplantation. 2002; 73: 193-197.
[13] Lee JM, Tu CF, Huang SC, Tsuji K, Chen RJ, Hu CY, Hsieh RP, Tai HC, Weng CN, Lee YC, Lee CJ. Attenuation of human-to-pig xenogenic cellular proliferation and Th1 response by expressing the human MHC II DQ exogenes on porcine cells. Transplant Proc. 2003; 35: 527-528.
[14] Liu J, Farmer JD Jr, Lane WS, Friedman J, Weissman I, Schreiber SL. Calcineurin is a common target of cyclophilin-cyclosporin A and FKBP-FK506 complexes. Cell. 1991; 66: 807-815.
[15] McKenna RM, Takemoto SK. Improving HLA matching for kidney transplantation by use of CREGs. Lancet. 2000; 355: 1842-1843.
[16] Mzali R, Seguin L, Liot C, Auger A, Pacaud P, Loirand G, Thibault C, Pierre J, Bertoglio J. Regulation of Rho signaling pathways in interleukin-2-stimulated human T-lymphocytes. FASEB J. 2005; 19: 1911-1913.
[17] Richter D, Reynolds SR, Harn DA. Candidate vaccine antigens that stimulate the cellular immune response of mice vaccinated with irradiated cercariae of Schistosoma mansoni. J Immunol. 1993; 151: 256-265.
[18] Sasaki H, Xu X-C, and Mohanakumar T. HLA-E and HLA-G expression on porcine endothelial cells inhibit xenoreactive human NK cells through CD94/NKG2-dependent and –independent pathways. J. Immunol., 1999. 163: 6301–6305.
[19] Schreiber SL. Chemistry and biology of the immunophilins and their immunosuppressive ligands. Science. 1991, 251: 283-287.
[20] Schreiber SL, Crabtree GR. The mechanism of action of cyclosporin A and FK506 Immunol Today. 1992; 13: 136-142.
[21] Sheldon S, Yonan NA, Aziz TN, Hasleton PS, Rahman AN, Deiraniya AK, Campbell CS, Dyer PA. The influence of histocompatibility on graft rejection and graft

survival within a single center population of heart transplant recipients. Transplantation. 1999; 68: 515-519.

[22] Starzl TE, Demetris AJ, Murase N, Ildstad S, Ricordi C, Trucco M. Cell migration, chimerism, and graft acceptance. Lancet. 1992; 339: 1579-1582.

[23] Sundberg EJ, Sawicki MW, Southwood S, Andersen PS, Sette A, Mariuzza RA. Minor structural changes in a mutated human melanoma antigen correspond to dramatically enhanced stimulation of a CD4+ tumor-infiltrating lymphocyte line. J .Mol. Biol. 2002, 319, 449–461.

[24] Tai HC, Ezzelarab M, Hara H, Ayares D, and Cooper DK. Progress in xenotransplantation following the introduction of gene-knockout technology. *Transpl Int*. 2007; 20:107-117.

[25] Tai HC, Tu CF, Lee JM, Ho LL, Tseng YL, Chou NK, Yang TS, Weng CN, Lee PH, Chang KJ, Tang YB. Long-term survival of HLA-DR15+ pig skin in SCID mice after reconstitution with human peripheral blood mononuclear cells and under short-term immunosuppression. Transplant Proc. 2008; 40: 570-573.

[26] Tsuji K, Hagihara M, Sato T, Shimura T, Takebe K, Munkhbat B. The role of HLA class II antigens/genes in xenogeneic iso, allo, and xeno transplantation. Transplant Proc. 1994; 26: 2441-2443.

[27] Tu CF, Hsieh SL, Lee JM, Yang LL, Sato T, Lee KH, Weng CN, Mao SJ, Tsuji K, Lee CJ. Successful generation of transgenic pigs for human decay-accelerating factor and human leucocyte antigen DQ. Transplant Proc. 2000; 32: 913-915.

[28] Tu CF, Lee JM, Sato T, Tai HC, Chung YF, Lee FR, Yang PW, Tsuji K, Lee CJ. Integration and expression of HLA-DR transgenic pigs. Xenoransplantation. 2001; 8 (Suppl. 1): 84.

[29] Tu CF, Lee JM, Sato T, Tai HC, Lee FR, Yang CK, Tsuji K, Lee CJ. Expression of HLA-DQ genes in transgenic pigs. Transplant Proc. 2003; 35: 513-515.

[30] Tu CF, Sato T, Hagihara M, Lee KH, Lee YC, Weng CN, Chu RM, Tsuji K, Lee CJ. Expression of HLA-DP antigen on peripheral blood mononuclear cells of HLA-DP transgenic pigs. Transplant Proc. 1998; 30: 3502-3503.

[31] Tu CF, Tai HC, Chen CM, Huang TT, Lee JM, Yang TS, Chen CH, Tseng YL, Chou NK, Lee PH. Human leukocyte antigen-DR matching improved skin graft survival from transgenic pigs to accommodate SCID mice reconstituted with human peripheral blood mononuclear cells. Transplant Proc. 2008; 40: 578-580.

[32] Tu CF, Tsuji K, Lee KH, Chu R, Sun TJ, Lee YC, Weng CN, Lee CJ. Generation of HLA-DP transgenic pigs for the study of xenotransplantation. Int Surg. 1999; 84: 176-182.

[33] Wang BT, Tu CF, Hsieh LJ, Tai HC, Chiu YL, Lee JM, Kuo SJ, Tsuji K, Lee CJ. Rapid detection of human HLA transgenes in pigs by fluorescence in situ hybridization (FISH) for adjuvant study of human xenotransplantation. *Xenotransplantation*. 2004; 11: 471-475.

[34] Weiss EH, Lilienfeld BG, Müller S, Müller E, Herbach N, Kessler B, Wanke R, Schwinzer R, Seebach JD, Wolf E, Brem G. HLA-E/human beta2-microglobulin transgenic pigs: protection against xenogeneic human anti-pig natural killer cell cytotoxicity. Transplantation. 2009; 87: 35-43.

[35] Woodside DG, Wooten DK, Teague TK, Miyamoto YJ, Caudell EG, Udagawa T, Andruss BF, McIntyre BW. Control of T lymphocyte morphology by the GTPase Rho. BMC Cell Biol. 2003; 4: 2.

5

Targeted Toxin as a Useful Reagent for Enrichment of α-Gal Epitope-Negative Cells Used for Somatic Cell Nuclear Transfer in Pigs

Masahiro Sato[1], Haiying Chi[2] and Kazuchika Miyoshi[2]
[1]*Section of Gene Expression Regulation, Frontier Science Research Center,*
[2]*Laboratory of Animal Reproduction, Faculty of Agriculture, Kagoshima University, Kagoshima*
Japan

1. Introduction

α-1,3-Galactosyltransferase (α-*GalT*) is a key enzyme in mediating the synthesis of the Galα1-3Gal (α-Gal) epitope on the cell surface of some mammalian species. Removal of the epitope is considered a prerequisite for xenotransplantation (Cooper et al., 1994). Thus, the production of genetically modified (GM) pigs that lack the expression of the α-Gal epitope has been the main target for pig-to-human xenotransplantation, and this can be performed by somatic cell nuclear transfer (SCNT) of porcine cells lacking α-*GalT* messenger RNA (mRNA) synthesis obtained by gene targeting (Lai et al., 2002; Dai et al., 2002; Phelps et al., 2003; Ramsoondar et al., 2003; Harrison et al., 2004; Kolber-Simonds et al., 2004; Takahagi et al., 2005). However, this approach is labor-intensive and time-consuming, and sometimes it is difficult to obtain knockout (KO) pigs. Other methods of genetically modifying pigs to obtain reduced levels of α-Gal epitope have been reported. One involves the production of cells/piglets overexpressing *Clostridium perfringens*-derived endo-β-galacosidase C (EndoGalC), which is capable of digesting α-Gal epitope (Yazaki et al., 2009; Himaki et al., 2010), and the other involves the production of cells/blastocysts overexpressing small interference RNA (siRNA) targeted to α-*GalT* mRNA (Yu et al., 2005; Zhu et al., 2005; Chi et al., 2010). Recently, zinc finger nuclease-mediated destruction of the endogenous α-*GalT* gene was reported by Hauschilda et al. (2011). In any case, however, for SCNT-mediated transgenesis, acquisition of a population of pure GM cells is a prerequisite because contamination of nontransfected cells or cells with low transgene expression would decrease the SCNT efficiency. Historically, cytotoxicity-based selection of α-Gal epitope-negative cells was first used for selection of cells completely lacking expression of *α-GalT* mRNA (Sharma et al., 2003). This can be performed by using specific antibodies (monoclonal antibodies) recognizing the α-Gal epitope and complement. Kolber-Simonds et al. (2004) used anti-α-Gal epitope antibodies from naive baboon plasma (natural antibodies) and baby rabbit complement. Baumann et al. (2004) also used a method similar to that of Kolber-Simonds et al. (2004). Although these cytotoxicity-based methods appear to be simple and convenient, it is often difficult to obtain α-Gal epitope-specific antibodies using these methods, and the strength of complement is sometimes variable, depending on the quality used. Fujimura et al. (2008) used magnet-activated cell sorting in the selection of α-Gal epitope-negative cells. This selection process successfully eliminates α-Gal epitope-positive cells by using biotin-labeled *Bandeiraea simplicifolia* isolectin-B_4 (IB4), a lectin that specifically binds to α-Gal epitope (Vaughan et al., 1994). However, in this case, contamination by a small number of α-Gal epitope-positive cells often occurs in the eluent after passage through the streptoavidin-conjugated column. Thus, Phelps et al. (2003) used a bacterial toxin, *Clostridium difficile* toxin A, which binds with high affinity to α-Gal epitope, to obtain *α-GalT*-deficient pig cells. This method appears very simple and easy to perform, except that the reagent itself is not always available, limiting its use.

We have recently proposed another approach for the elimination of α-Gal epitope-positive cells. This approach is called targeted toxin technology (http://www.ATSbio.com), with which α-Gal epitope-expressing cells can be efficiently eliminated by incubation of target cells in the presence of toxin-labeled IB4. This selection procedure is rapid and simple because α-Gal epitope-expressing porcine cells are rapidly removed after incubation with toxin-labeled IB4 for 1–2 h at 37°C and subsequent cultivation in normal medium for more than 10 days, as will be described later in more detail.

Targeted toxins consist of the ribosome-inactivating protein saporin (Stirpe et al., 1992), which is conjugated to a target molecule that recognizes a cell-specific marker. When the conjugate is administered to cells of interest, it binds to the target cells and is absorbed, releasing saporin, which inactivates ribosomes. Cells not expressing the target molecule do not bind or absorb the conjugate, and are not affected. This can be performed simply by co-incubating target cells with the targeted toxins for a short period before culture in normal conditions, as described previously. It does not require additional treatment, such as that with a complement to kill target cells, and the targeted toxins themselves are commercially available from Advanced Targeting Systems Inc. (San Diego, CA, USA). When the targeted toxin is not available, it is possible to form a complex between saporin and the molecule of interest (which must be expressed on the cell surface) by hand. In this context, targeted toxins are useful as a powerful tool for removing unwanted cells from a pool of GM cells. In fact, negative selection using targeted toxins has already been proven useful in vivo (Wiley and Kline, 2000; Vulchanova et al., 2001; Tarpley et al., 2004) and in vitro (Akasaka et al., 2010).

In our previous experiments (Akasaka et al., 2010), we demonstrated that porcine embryonic fibroblasts (PEFs) expressing the EndoGalC gene strongly can survive after treatment with IB4 conjugated with saporin (hereafter referred to as IB4-SAP), but those that do so weakly or not at all died within 3 or 4 days after the treatment. When the surviving cells were inspected for possible expression of α-Gal epitope on their cell surface using fluorescence-labeled IB4, no distinct fluorescence was noted, indicating the success of the targeted toxin technology.

2. Results and perspective

In this review, we demonstrate another successful attempt performed in our laboratory of enriching porcine cells with highly reduced amounts of α-Gal epitope. First, the PEFs were transfected with the siRNA expression vector pPNER5 (Fig. 1A), which carries enhanced green fluorescent protein (*EGFP*) cDNA and neomycin resistance gene (*neo*) expression units, together with an siRNA fragment targeted to the middle region of α-*GalT* mRNA (Chi et al., in press). We expected that the PEFs stably transfected with the pPNER5 plasmid would exhibit EGFP-derived fluorescence but decreased the expression of α-Gal epitope on their cell surface. Staining of transfected cells cultured for 10 days without drug selection with Alexa Fluor 594 (red fluorescence)-labeled IB4 revealed that approximately 64% of fluorescent cells (132 cells counted in total) were less distinctly stained with lectin (arrows in Fig. 1D-a–c). The image analysis of these cells demonstrated 60–95% reduction in the level of α-Gal epitope expressed in the normal cells. However, the remaining fluorescent cells were distinctly stained with lectin (arrowheads in Fig. 1D-d–f), suggesting silencing or low levels of siRNA expression from the integrated pPNER5 plasmid. To eliminate these fluorescent cells (but still expressing the α-Gal epitope) and nonfluorescent cells (probably nontransfected cells), the cells were treated with IB4-SAP (1 × 10^6 cells; 10 days after transfection). Inspection of the cells 1 day after the treatment revealed massive cell death in the IB4-SAP-treated group (Fig. 1C-a) but not in the control group (SAP alone; Fig. 1C-b), indicating the effectiveness of IB4-SAP in killing α-Gal epitope-expressing cells. Four days after the IB4-SAP treatment, the cells were passaged from a 30-mm dish onto a 60-mm dish and cultured in the absence of a selection drug for approximately 2 weeks. The number of colonies generated ranged 1–5. These colonies were next picked up by a paper method (Nakayama et al., 2007) and propagated systematically. Of the 3 colonies tested, all exhibited bright green fluorescence but reduced levels of α-Gal epitope expression on their cell surface, as evidenced by the staining with Alexa Fluor 594-labeled IB4 (Fig. 1D-g–i). We next performed SCNT using the IB4-SAP-treated pPNER5 transfectants. Out of 154 enucleated oocytes reconstituted with pPNER5-PEFs, the developing blastocysts exhibited bright green fluorescence around an embryo (Fig. 2A-b, e), suggesting success of the SCNT. Staining the blastocyst derived from the SCNT of the pPNER5-PEFs with Alexa Fluor 594-labeled IB4 demonstrated a great decrease in fluorescence on its cell surface (Fig. 2A-c). This was in contrast with the blastocyst derived from the SCNT of the pEGFP-N1-PEFs (Nakayama et al., 2007), which exhibited extensive staining with lectin (Fig. 2A-f). Reverse transcription-polymerase chain reaction (RT-PCR) analysis demonstrated that all of the tested samples (5/5 tested) exhibited complete loss of the target 586-base pair (bp) band corresponding to the endogenous *α-GalT* mRNA (lanes 1–5 in Fig. 2B). In contrast, all (2/2 tested) of the SCNT blastocysts derived from eggs reconstituted with pEGFP-N1-PEF nuclei exhibited a clear band of 586 bp (lanes 8 and 9 in Fig. 2B). These data indicate the effectiveness of RNA interference (RNAi) in the SCNT-derived porcine embryos and suggest the usefulness of IB4-SAP for enrichment of porcine cells with highly reduced levels of α-Gal epitope prior to SCNT-mediated production of GM piglets suitable for pig-to-human xenotransplantation.

Our major concern is how long this RNAi-mediated suppression of endogenous *α-GalT* mRNA will continue beyond the blastocyst stage. Therefore, it is required to transfer the SCNT blastocysts into recipients for obtaining cloned GM fetuses or animals that have been carried to term in which reduced levels of α-Gal epitope expression are expected to be maintained.

In conclusion, we demonstrate the usefulness of targeted toxin technology here, using IB4-SAP for enriching GM porcine cells in which α-Gal epitope synthesis is almost suppressed. These enriched cells are useful for cell transplantation or for SCNT-mediated generation of GM pigs that are optimized for xenotransplantation.

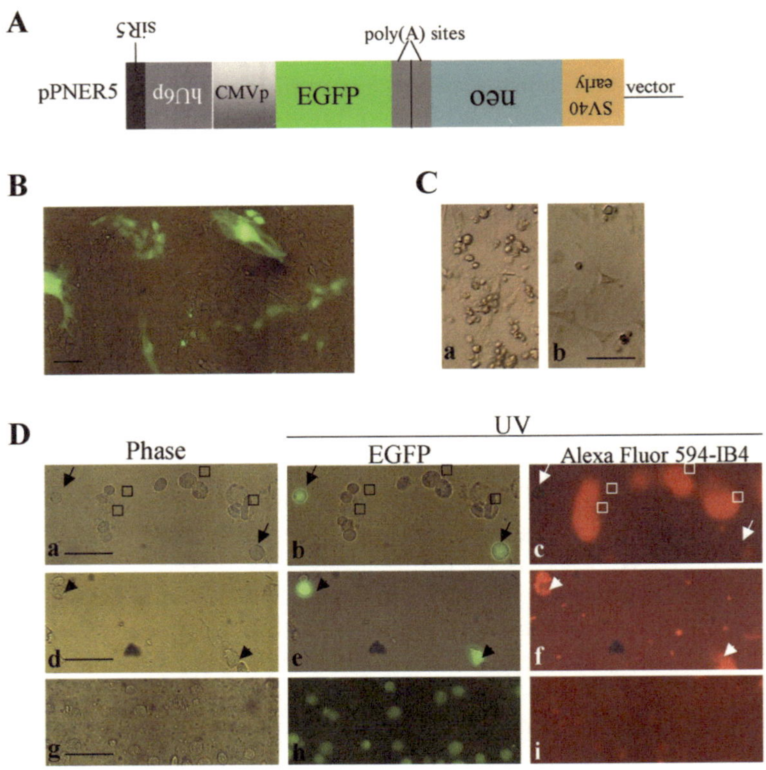

Fig. 1. A. Plasmid pPNER5 constructed by inserting a siRNA expression unit (comprising hU6p and siR5) upstream of the cytomegalovirus promoter (CMVp) in pEGFP-N1 plasmid. Abbreviations: EGFP, enhanced green fluorescent protein cDNA; neo, neomycin resistance gene; siR5, siRNA targeted to *α-GalT* mRNA; SV40 early, SV40 enhancer and early promoter; hU6p, human U6 promoter. B. EGFP expression in pPNER5-transfected PEFs cultured in G418-free PEF medium for 10 days after transfection. Approximately 10% of the cells were observed to express EGFP-derived green fluorescence. Bar = 25 μm. C. Cells 1 day after treatment with pPNER5-PEFs with IB4-SAP (a) or control SAP alone (b). Before dish-washing, a number of floating cells are visible in the IB4-SAP-treated dish (a) but almost none in the control dish (b). Bar = 25 μm. D. Cytochemical staining with IB4 lectin. a–f, Cells 10 days after transfection with linearized pPNER5 plasmid stained with Alexa Fluor 594-labeled IB4 lectin. Note that the fluorescent cells exhibit a mosaic pattern for lectin staining, indicating a mixture of cells expressing (indicated by arrowheads in d–f), not expressing, or weakly expressing α-Gal epitope (indicated by arrows in a–c). In contrast, untransfected nonfluorescent PEFs exhibit strong red fluorescence on the cell surface (denoted by quadrants in a–c). g–i, Cells surviving for 1 month after IB4-SAP treatment were examined for the presence of α-Gal epitope on their surfaces by Alexa Fluor 594-labeled IB4. As expected, almost all the cells treated with IB4-SAP were slightly or not at all stained with lectin. Phase, microphotographs taken under light; UV, microphotographs taken under UV + light. Bar = 25 μm.

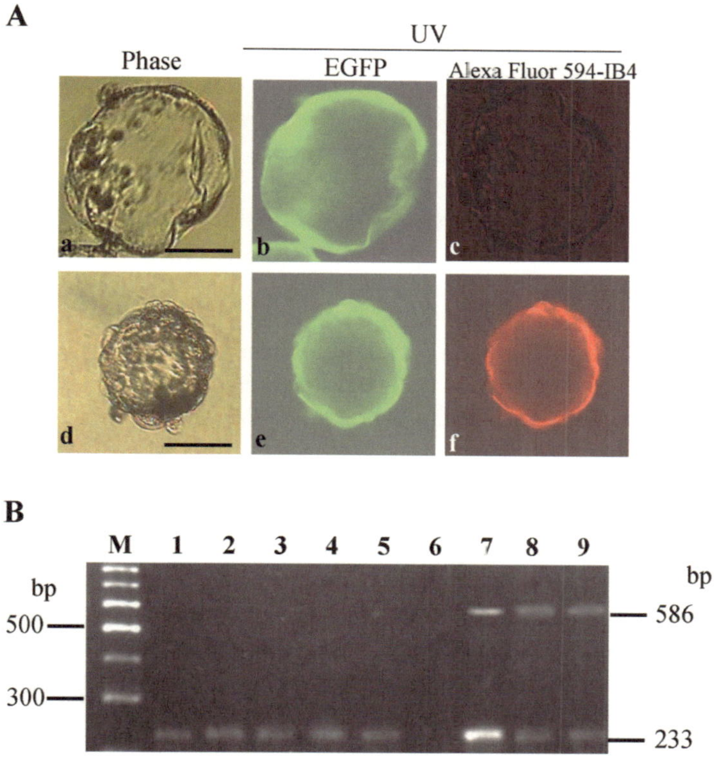

Fig. 2. A. a–c, Reduced expression of α-Gal epitope in blastocysts derived from oocytes reconstituted with the pPNER5-PEFs. Developing SCNT blastocysts were stained with Alexa Fluor 594-labeled IB4 before observation using a fluorescence microscope. Note the bright green fluorescence around the whole embryo (b) but marked reduction in red fluorescence on its cell surface (c). d–f, Control blastocyst derived from the oocytes reconstituted with the control pEGFP-N1-PEFs. Note the bright green (e) and red (f) fluorescence around the embryo. Phase, microphotographs taken under light; UV, microphotographs taken under UV + light. Scale bar = 50 μm. B. RT-PCR analysis of endogenous *α-GalT* and *β-actin* mRNA in blastocysts derived from oocytes reconstituted with pPNER5-PEFs. Lanes 1–5, Blastocysts derived from oocytes reconstituted with pPNER5-transfected PEFs; lane 6, water subjected to RT-PCR (negative control); lane 7, PEFs (positive control); lanes 8 and 9, blastocysts derived from oocytes reconstituted with control pEGFP-N1-PEFs.

3. References

Akasaka, E.; Watanabe, S.; Himaki, T.; Ohtsuka, M.; Yoshida, M.; Miyoshi, K.; Sato, M. (2010). Enrichment of xenograft-competent genetically modified pig cells using a targeted toxin, isolectin BS-I-B4 conjugate. *Xenotransplantation*, 17: 81-89

Baumann, BC.; Forte, P.; Hawley, RJ.; Rieben, R.; Schneider, MK.; Seebach, JD. (2004). Lack of galactose-α-1,3-galactose expression on porcine endothelial cells prevents complement-induced lysis but not direct xenogeneic NK cytotoxicity. *J Immunol*, 172: 6460-6467

Chi, H.; Shinohara, M.; Yokomine, T.; Sato, M.; Takao, S.; Yoshida, M.; Miyoshi, K. Successful suppression of endogenous α-1,3-galactosyltransferase expression by RNA interference in pig embryos generated in vitro. *J Reprod Dev*, (in press).

Cooper, DK.; Koren, E.; Oriol, R. (1994). Oligosaccharides and discordant xenotransplantation. *Immunol Rev*, 141: 31-58

Dai, Y.; Vaught, TD.; Boone, J.; Chen, SH.; Phelps, CJ.; Ball, S.; Monahan, JA.; Jobst, PM.; McCreath, KJ.; Lamborn, AE.; Cowell-Lucero, JL.; Wells, KD.; Colman, A.; Polejaeva, IA.; Ayares, DL. (2002). Targeted disruption of the alpha1,3-galactosyltransferase gene in cloned pigs. *Nat Biotechnol*, 20: 251-255

Fujimura, T.; Takahagi, Y.; Shigehisa, T.; Nagashima, H.; Miyagawa, S.; Shirakura, R.; Murakami, H. (2008). Production of α1,3-galactosyltransferase gene-deficient pigs by somatic cell nuclear transfer: a novel selection method for galα1,3-Gal antigen-deficient cells. *Mol Reprod Dev*, 75: 1372-1378

Harrison, S.; Boquest, A.; Grupen, C.; Faast, R.; Guildolin, A.; Giannakis, C.; Crocker, L.; McIlfatrick, S.; Ashman, R.; Wengle, J.; Lyons, I.; Tolstoshev, P.; Cowan, P.; Robins, A.; O'Connell, P.; D'Apice, AJ.; Nottle M. (2004). An efficient method for producing alpha(1,3)-galactosyltransferase gene knockout pigs. *Cloning Stem Cells*, 6: 327-331

Hauschilda, J.; Petersena, B.; Santiago, Y.; Queissera, A.; Carnwatha, JW.; Lucas-Hahna, A.; Zhang, L.; Meng, X.; Gregory, PD.; Schwinzerd, R.; Cost, GJ.; Niemann, H. (2011). Efficient generation of a biallelic knockout in pigs using zinc-finger nucleases. *Proc Natl Acad Sci USA*, 108: 12013-12017

Himaki, T.; Watanabe, S.; Chi, H.; Yoshida, M.; Miyoshi, K.; Sato, M. (2010). Production of genetically modified porcine blastocysts by somatic cell nuclear transfer: preliminary results toward production of xenograft-competent miniature pigs. *J Reprod Dev*, 56: 630-638

Kolber-Simonds, D.; Lai, L.; Watt, SR.; Denaro, M.; Arn, S.; Augenstein, ML.; Betthauser, J.; Carter, DB.; Greenstein, JL.; Hao, Y.; Im, GS.; Liu, Z.; Mell, GD.; Murphy, CN.; Park, KW.; Rieke, A.; Ryan, DJ.; Sachs, DH.; Forsberg, EJ.; Prather, RS.; Hawley, RJ. (2004). Production of alpha-1,3-galactosyltransferase null pigs by means of nuclear transfer with fibroblasts bearing loss of heterozygosity mutations. *Proc Natl Acad Sci USA*, 101: 7335-7340

Lai, L.; Kolber-Simonds, D.; Park, KW.; Cheong, HT.; Greenstein, JL.; Im, GS.; Samuel, M.; Bonk, A.; Rieke, A.; Day, BN.; Murphy, CN.; Carter, DB.; Hawley, RJ.; Prather, RS.

(2002). Production of alpha-1,3-galactosyltransferase knockout pigs by nuclear transfer cloning. *Science*, 295: 1089-1092

Nakayama, A.; Sato, M.; Shinohara, M.; Matsubara, S.; Yokomine, T.; Akasaka, E.; Yoshida, M.; Takao S. (2007). Efficient transfection of primarily cultured porcine embryonic fibroblasts using the Amaxa nucleofection system™. *Cloning Stem Cells*, 9: 523-534

Phelps, CJ.; Koike, C.; Vaught, TD.; Boone, J.; Wells, KD.; Chen, SH.; Ball, S.; Specht, SM.; Polejaeva, IA.; Monahan, JA.; Jobst, PM.; Sharma, SB.; Lamborn, AE.; Garst, AS.; Moore, M.; Demetris, AJ.; Rudert, WA.; Bottino, R.; Bertera, S.; Trucco, M.; Starzl, TE.; Dai, Y.; Ayares, DL. (2003). Production of alpha 1,3-galactosyltransferase-deficient pigs. *Science*, 299: 411-414

Ramsoondar, JJ.; Machy, Z.; Costa, C.; Williams, BL.; Fodor, WL.; Bondioli, KR. (2003). Production of alpha 1,3-galactosyltransferase-knockout cloned pigs expressing human alpha 1,2-fucosylosyltransferase. *Biol Reprod*, 69: 437-445

Sharma, A.; Naziruddin, B.; Cui, C.; Martin, MJ.; Xu, H.; Wan, H.; Lei, Y.; Harrison, C.; Yin, J.; Okabe, J.; Mathews, C.; Stark, A.; Adams, CS.; Houtz, J.; Wiseman, BS.; Byrne, GW.; Logan, JS. (2003). Pig cells that lack the gene forα1-3 galactosyltransferase express low levels of the gal antigen. *Transplantation*, 75: 430-436

Stirpe, F.; Barbieri, L.; Battelli, MG.; Soria, M.; Lappi, DA. (1992). Ribosome-inactivating proteins from plants: present status and future prospects. *Biotechnology*, 10: 405-412

Takahagi, Y.; Fujimura, T.; Miyagawa, S.; Nagashima, H.; Shigehisa, T.; Shirakura, R.; Murakami, H. (2005). Production of alpha 1,3-galactosyltransferase gene knockout pigs expressing both human decay-accelerating factor and *N*-acetylglucosaminyltransferase III. *Mol Reprod Dev*, 71: 331-338

Tarpley, JW.; Martin G Kohler, MG.; Martin, WJ. (2004). The behavioral and neuroanatomical effects of IB4-saporin treatment in rat models of nociceptive and neuropathic pain. *Brain Res*, 1029: 65-76

Vaughan, HA.; Loveland, BE.; Sandrin MS. (1994). Gal(α1-3)Gal is the major xenoepitope expressed on pig endothelial cells recognized by naturally occurring cytotoxic human antibodies. *Transplantation*, 58: 879-882

Vulchanova, L.; Olson, TH.; Stone, LS.; Riedl, MS.; Elde, R.; Honda, CN. (2001). Cytotoxic targeting of isolectin IB4-binding sensory neurons. *Neuroscience*, 108: 143-155

Wiley, RG.; Kline IV, RH. (2000). Neuronal lesioning with axonally transported toxins. J *Neurosci Methods*, 103: 73-82

Yazaki, S.; Iwamoto, M.; Onishi, A.; Miwa, Y.; Suzuki, S.; Fuchimoto, D.; Sembon, S.; Furusawa, T.; Hashimoto, M.; Oishi, T.; Liu, D.; Nagasaka, T.; Kuzuya, T.; Maruyama, S.; Ogawa, H.; Kadomatsu, K.; Uchida, K.; Nakao, A.; Kobayashi, T. (2009). Successful cross-breeding of cloned pigs expressing endo-beta-galactosidase C and human decay accelerating factor. *Xenotransplantation*, 16: 511-521

Yu, L.; Miao, H.; Guo, L. (2005). Effect of RNA inhibition on Gal alpha-1,3-Gal expression in PIEC cells. *DNA Cell Biol*, 24: 235-243

Zhu, M.; Xia, ZX.; Wang, SS.; Cao, RH.; Qi, HG.; Chen, D.; Liu, B.; Zhang, WJ.; Chen, S. (2005). The role RNA inhibition of alpha-1,3-GT plays in resistance to complement mediated cytotoxicity of pig endothelial cells. *Zhonghua Yi Xue Za Zhi*, 85: 1133-1136

Part 3

Clinic and Preclinic

6

Developing Xenostandards for Microbiological Safety: New Zealand Experience

O. Garkavenko, S. Wynyard, D. Nathu and R. Elliott
Living Cell Technologies
New Zealand

1. Introduction

Human patients have the potential to become infected with animal viruses following xenotransplantation. Concerns have also been raised that in a worst case scenario, pathogens originating from pig donors may adapt and then propagate to the wider public resulting in a new epidemic (Fiane, Mollnes, & Degre, 2000; Fishman, 2001a; Onions et al., 2000; Patience, Wilkinson, & Weiss, 1997; Weiss, 2003). The likelihood that cross-species infection may occur is enhanced in a xenotransplantation setting because normal host defences such as skin and mucosal surfaces are bypassed and direct contact between donor and recipient cells is maintained for extended periods of time (O'Rourke, 2000). Similarly for applications that use immunosuppression to prevent xenograft rejection, host complement-mediated immunity is circumvented (Takeuchi, Magre & Patience, 2005). Currently pigs are recognised as the most popular choice as donor animals due in part to their ostensibly lower infectious risk (compared with non-human primates), excellent breeding potential, comparable organ size, physiological similarity, amenability to genetic modification, non contentious public perception and the relatively moderate costs associated with their maintenance (Sachs, Sykes, Robson, & Cooper, 2001). In terms of pig pathogens it has been determined that the preponderance of fungi, bacteria and parasites can be excluded as major risk factors simply by the use of good animal husbandry practices in Specific Pathogen Free (SPF) herds (Ye, Niekrasz, Kosanke, Welsh, Jordan et al, 1994). Consequently viruses are recognised as the predominant infectious agent for zoonosis owing to their rapid rate of evolution and excellent adaptive competence within new hosts. Precedents for cross-species infection of viruses and adaptation in humans are numerous and include several notorious examples, notably AIDS (Gao, Bailes, Robertson, Chen, Rodenburg et al, 1999) and avian influenza [reviewed in (Alexander & Brown, 2000)]. Although pigs are not always a natural reservoir for exogenous viruses, it has been hypothesised that swine may act as "mixing vessels" for adaptation to human hosts, as is certainly the case for avian viruses such as Severe Acute Respiratory Syndrome (SARS) (Bush, 2004).

Recommendations to minimize cross-species infection stipulate that donor pigs should be maintained in quarantined facilities and monitored for the presence of exogenous pathogens. This type of program requires significant resources so there is considerable incentive to monitor only those viruses that are relevant. Several comprehensive reviews have been published describing zoonotic agents in pigs that may potentially cause disease in transplant recipients and theoretically the population at large (Fishman, 2001a, 2001b; Mueller, Takeuchi, Mattiuzzo, & Scobie, 2011; Scobie & Takeuchi, 2009; Takeuchi et al, 2005). A particularly valuable resource is the report in the journal Xenotransplantation by Shuurman (2009) that offers a consensus view of organisms that should be excluded from donor pigs. The most important pathogens are reported to be swine influenza viruses belonging to the influenza A genus, Nipah virus, *Marburgvirus* and *Ebolavirus* of the *Filoviridae* family, rotaviruses, parvoviruses, hepatitis E and herpesviruses such as porcine circovirus type 2 (PCV2) and porcine lymphotrophic herpes virus type 2 (PLHV2).

In New Zealand a very deliberate strategy was employed in order to maximise patient safety by ensuring that these viruses and other pathogens were absent in a donor herd destined for clinical trials. Two important goals were considered integral to the success of the New Zealand approach. The first goal was to ensure the safety of donor material and was achieved by utilising the following steps: (1) investigating the health status of the New Zealand pig population; (2) developing and implementing an algorithm for herd selection; (3) establishing a program to characterise pig endogenous retrovirus; (4) defining a testing schedule to maintain the specific pathogen-free (SPF) status of the donor herd; (5) certifying the health of all donor animals and (6) certifying the safety of the final product. The second goal required the implementation of a robust monitoring program for patient follow-up post-transplant. In this case specific emphasis was placed upon the development of reliable and sensitive assays to detect pig pathogens in humans as well as developing a network of collaborative reference laboratories. Important also was the establishment of a xeno-microbiology laboratory and its accreditation as a medical diagnostic laboratory to guarantee the highest diagnostic standards. Using this strategy regulatory approval was obtained to begin the first clinical trials using insulin-producing cells (DIABECELL®) for the treatment of Type I Diabetes (http://www.lctglobal.com/lctdiabecell-diabetes-treatment.php).

2. Determining infections relevant to xenotransplantation in NZ

The Public Health Service Guidelines on Infectious Disease Issues in Xenotransplantation states that monitoring programs for source animals should be tailored to specific geographical areas (U.S Food and Drug [FDA], 2001). This recommendation implies knowledge of the local pig infection profile and in particular, knowledge of virus infections potentially relevant to xenotransplantation. The health status of the NZ pig population is considered to be favourable thanks largely to its geographic remoteness and strict animal health control policies. Unlike many countries NZ remains free from infectious vesicular diseases such as foot and mouth, vesicular stomatitis and vesicular exanthema. Notable infections like rabies, Brucella suis, swine fever, pseudorabies and spongiform encephalopathy are also absent. Routine screening protocols for a source herd intended for xenotransplantation may encompass up to 45 different pathogens (H. J. Schuurman, 2009) many of which are common to veterinary practices. However, for the NZ pig population very limited data was initially available regarding viruses such as Porcine Cytomegalovirus (PCMV), Porcine Lymphotrophic Herpesvirus (PLHV), Encephalomyocarditis Virus (EMCV), Porcine Circovirus Virus (PCV) and pig Hepatitis E Virus (HEV). In order to extend the data regarding the prevalence of these potentially zoonotic viruses an investigatory screening program was performed that tested representatives from herds throughout NZ (Garkavenko, Elliott, & Croxson, 2005; Garkavenko, Muzina, et al., 2004; Garkavenko et al., 2001). This information led to a significantly improved understanding of the infection profile within NZ pig breeds and facilitated the development of a screening protocol for viruses that were particularly relevant to xenotransplantation. Numerous NZ pig herds intended as a source of islet cells for transplantation were comprehensively assessed according to this screening protocol.

Having established the epidemiology of our test panel of viruses in NZ pigs, a further examination was performed in one-week old piglets (the donor age group from which islet cells are harvested). All one-week-old piglets were free of the majority of tested viruses. This finding implies that infection with PCMV, PLHV and HEV takes place peri- or post-natal and that despite the presence of infection within a herd, new-born piglets and their tissues may remain virus-free. This conclusion is in contrast with another study in which the PLHV virus was shown to be vertically transmitted although it should be noted that this type of transmission phenomenon is considered to be a rare event (Tucker et al., 2003). The presence of PCV2 in tissues and faecal samples of one-week-old piglets was an unexpected result. Although it was shown that this virus can be transmitted vertically (Bogdan et al., 2001.; Ladekjaer-Mikkelson et al., 2001; O'Connor et al., 2001; Sanchez, Nauwynck, McNeilly, Allan, & Pensaert, 2001), there is a common view that this virus is associated with severe pathology in new-born piglets, and its vertical transmission is also a rare event.

Three factors must be considered when assessing the infectious risk of PCV2 associated with xenotransplantation: (1) the ubiquity of the PCV type 2 virus (Celera & Carasova, 2002; Garkavenko et al., 2005; Kim et al., 2002; Labarque, Nauwynck, Mesu, & Pesaert, 2000; Trujano, Iglesias, Segales, & Palacios, 2001; Wattrang et al., 2002); (2) the potential that the virus might be transmitted vertically without showing any sign of abnormality (Garkavenko, Croxson, et al., 2004) and (3) transmission of the virus occurs in human cells *in vitro* (Hattermann, 2002, unpublished data), and in experimental mice *in vivo* (Kiupel et al., 2001). Despite evidence that caesarean section and barrier rearing techniques are effective in excluding PCV and PLHV from pig populations, these interventions do not guarantee the exclusion of all viruses from a pig herd (Tucker et al., 2003). While each of these factors requires further intensive study, it seems reasonable to suggest that any source herd intended for xenotransplantation must be free from PCV and PLHV.

3. Selection criteria for xenotransplantation donors

The microbiological 'xenostandard' demands the absence of identifiable infectious agents in the source herd. A NZ donor herd that fulfilled this standard was found through a monitoring program that required the completion of several key tasks. This included a viral profile assessment of the pig population within the country, identification of a specific source herd, development of safety criteria including a plan to manage positive animals and finally, implementation of a multilevel monitoring schedule encompassing pig founders through to the final product. For the New Zealand herd an algorithm to determine whether source animals were suitable for xenotransplantation was developed (see Figure 1). This algorithm stipulates that if an agent capable of infecting human cells cannot be eradicated from the herd then an assessment of risk versus benefit must be made. Using this algorithm it became apparent that pigs from the Auckland Islands (AI) represented the ideal donor herd.

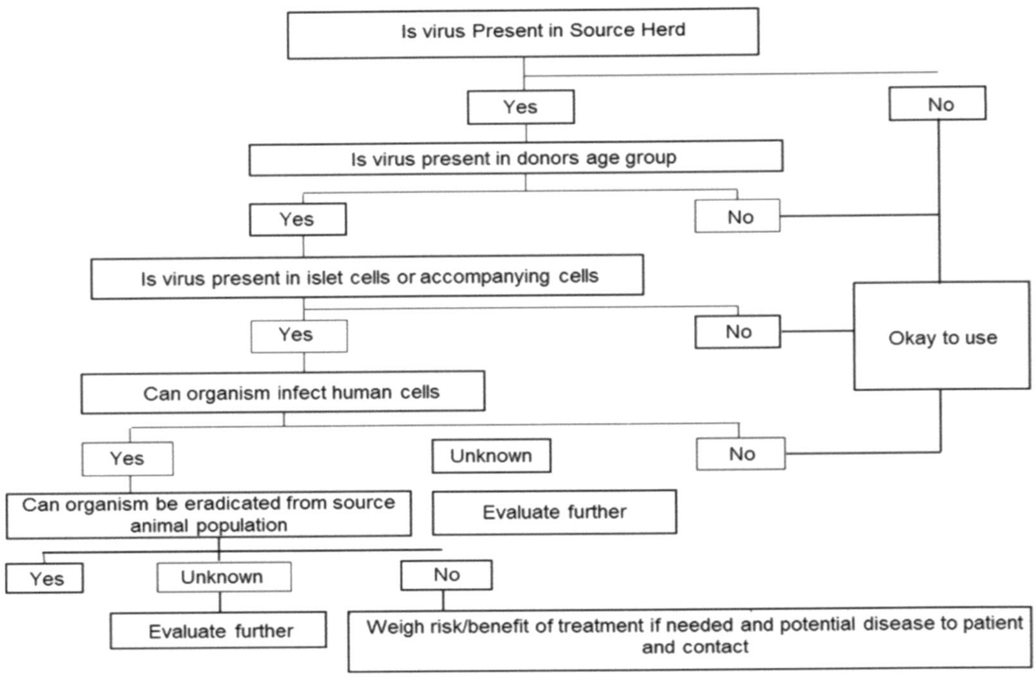

Fig. 1. Algorithm for donor herd selection

3.1 The Auckland Island donor herd

The Auckland Islands are a group of islands to the south of mainland New Zealand. In 1807 individual pigs were first introduced to the island as a source of food for whalers and shipwrecked sailors. Over subsequent decades these animals were reported to be thriving leading to further releases in 1840, 1842 and 1890. By the end of the nineteenth century a strong feral pig population had been established that was to remain isolated for the next hundred years. By the mid 1990's these animals were marked for eradication by the New Zealand Department of Conservation as part of a program to restore the natural ecosystems on the island. Consequently the Rare Breeds Conservation Society of New Zealand (RBCSNZ) attempted to preserve the breed in captivity. In 1999 a RBCSNZ expedition caught and removed seventeen pigs, including several pregnant sows, from Auckland Island, transferring them to Invercargill, New Zealand. These animals were subsequently acquired by the private biotech company Living Cell Technologies for the purposes of providing donor material for cell transplantation in humans for the treatment of disease. Currently these animals are maintained within quarantined facilities with one founder herd of approximately 40 animals kept in Invercargill, New Zealand and a second smaller donor herd of 15 animals located in Kumeu, Auckland, New Zealand. These animals as well as the cellular products derived from them are subject to a rigorous testing schedule for an extensive list of pathogens (Table 1).

Pathogen/Disease	Type	Frequency	NZ Status	Herd Status
Porcine Circovirus Type 1	Virus	Quarterly	Ubiquitous	Absent
Porcine Circovirus Type 2	DNA virus	Annually	Not present	Absent
Porcine Lymphotrophic Herpesvirus Type 2	DNA virus	Quarterly	Ubiquitous	Absent
Porcine Cytomegalovirus	DNA virus	Quarterly	Ubiquitous	Absent
Toxoplasma gondii	Parasitic protozoan	As Required	Ubiquitous	Absent
Porcine Hepatitis E virus	RNA virus	Annually	Ubiquitous	Absent
Rotavirus	RNA virus	Annually	Ubiquitous	Absent
Reovirus	RNA virus	Annually	Ubiquitous	Absent
Porcine Enterovirus Type 1	RNA virus	Annually	Ubiquitous	Absent
Porcine Enterovirus Type 3	RNA virus	Annually	Ubiquitous	Absent
Porcine Encephalomyocarditis Virus	RNA virus	Annually	Ubiquitous	Absent
Mycoplasma hyopneumoniae	Bacterium	Annually	Ubiquitous	Absent
Bovine Virus Diarrhea	RNA virus	Annually	Ubiquitous	Absent
Aujesky's Disease	RNA virus	Annually	Not present	Absent
Porcine Parvovirus	DNA virus	Quarterly	Ubiquitous	Absent
Porcine Reproductive and Respiratory Syndrome Virus	RNA virus	Annually	Not present	Absent
Leptospira hardjo	Bacterium	Quarterly	Ubiquitous	Absent
Leptospira pomona	Bacterium	Quarterly	Ubiquitous	Absent
Leptospira tarrasovi	Bacterium	Quarterly	Ubiquitous	Absent
Campylobacter	Bacterium	Annually	Ubiquitous	Absent
Coccidia (Isospora)	Parasitic protozoan	Annually	Ubiquitous	Absent
Cryptosporidium	Parasitic protozoan	Annually	Ubiquitous	Absent
Yersinia	Bacterium	Annually	Ubiquitous	Absent
E.coli K88	Bacterium	Annually	Ubiquitous	Absent
Salmonella	Bacterium	Annually	Ubiquitous	Absent

Table 1. List of pathogens tested for in the NZ Auckland Island donor herd.

3.2 Multilevel monitoring

A key facet of the 'selection algorithm' is that a multilevel monitoring process is adopted that begins with the regular screening (see table 1) of every individual pig within the donor herd. For certain pathogens such as PCV2, PLHV2 and PCMV sampling maybe performed from multiple tissues including pancreas and peripheral blood leukocytes (PBL). In the case of HEV both blood serum and faeces are processed. This is followed by the screening of all the sows' pre and post farrowing as well as the screening of each piglet donor (see table 2 for tests performed). Prior to surgery and removal of organs each piglet is examined for signs of infection. Any abnormalities are noted and in certain cases further consultation maybe sort from veterinary specialists. A strict policy is enforced to exclude even slightly suspect piglets from contributing donor material. Following removal of donor material each piglet is subject to a full post mortem by veterinary pathologists. Lastly the transplant product itself is screened immediately prior to transplantation. This final clearance is mandatory before the product can be released for transplantation. Such a comprehensive schedule of testing was judged necessary to assure the microbiological safety of xenografts and to satisfy NZ regulatory authorities.

Sows (pre- and post-farrowing)	Piglets	Injected product
Leptospira	HEV	Toxoplasma PCR
PPV	Toxoplasma serology	PCV2
Mycoplasma	Post-mortem autopsy	PLHV
Toxoplasma	PCV2*	PCMV
HEV	PLHV2*	HEV
PLHV	PCMV*	Mycoplasma
PCV2		
PCMV		

Table 2. List of porcine microorganisms for multi-level screening program. *PCR is performed on DNA extracted from both peripheral blood leukocytes and pancreas tissue.

4. Porcine Endogenous Retrovirus (PERV) – Developing a standard approach

In comparison to exogenous viruses a unique problem is posed by endogenous retroviruses (ERV). In pigs this pathogen is known as Porcine Endogenous Retrovirus (PERV) and is ubiquitous to all pig species studied to date. Endogenous retroviruses can be distinguished from exogenous types by their presence as genomic components that do not present pathology in their natural host (Stoye, Le Tissier, Takeuchi, Patience, & Weiss, 1998). Moreover, endogenous retroviruses behave like normal cellular genes in that they are inherited by the offspring and not acquired by infection. Accordingly PERV cannot be removed by conventional barrier methods instead requiring more elaborate strategies such as the selective breeding of pigs with favourable PERV genetic characteristics (Garkavenko, Wynyard, Nathu, Muzina, Muzina et al, 2008; Garkavenko, Wynyard, Nathu, Simond, Muzina et al, 2008; Stoye et al, 1998), or the development of vaccines to protect against PERV transmission or the inhibition of PERV expression by RNA interference using PERV-specific short hairpin RNA (shRNA) and retroviral vectors [reviewed in (Denner, 2008)]. Like most retroviruses PERV has an element of unpredictability in regards to its transmission potential. The concern exists that retroviral transmission may occur 'silently' by means of an undetectable recombination event, oncogenesis or alteration in gene regulation resulting in pathology that does not manifest until decades later. Such transmission is typical for gammaretroviruses and xenotransplantation could provide the right environment for selection of variants that can efficiently infect the human population. Numerous studies have been performed examining the risk of PERV transmission as it relates to xenotransplantation with the consensus that PERV must be considered an endogenous agent to be reduced or excluded where possible in animals destined for clinical use (H.J. Schuurman & Pierson, 2008; Taylor, 2008; Wilson, 2008).

4.1 PERV infectivity *in vitro* – The gold standard

With regard to PERV infectious characteristics, a standard infectivity method can be applied to check the infectivity of primary tissues such as peripheral blood mononuclear cells (PBMC) and islets derived from SPF pigs (Patience, Wilkinson, et al., 1997; Takeuchi et al., 1998). Such data is necessary because PCR for either the PERV *pol* or PERV *env* region does not always provide information on the transmission characteristics of PERV. In fact recombinant PERV is most often detected in transmission studies by co-culturing primary pig cells with target human cell lines as was performed in the NZ SPF herd. To ensure the release of infectious PERV particles (if any), tested cells were mitogenically stimulated prior to co-culture with standard susceptible cell lines 293 (to elucidate xeno-tropic PERV) and St-Iowa (to elucidate eco-tropic PERV). Although mitogenic stimulation enhanced proliferation of all tested cells, no evidence of PERV transmission was detected in the infectivity test with both human and pig target cells using PBMC or islet cells isolated from the New Zealand SPF pigs (Garkavenko, Wynyard, Nathu, Muzina, et al., 2008; Garkavenko, Wynyard, Nathu, Simond, et al., 2008). Thus it was concluded that the New Zealand SPF pigs could be classified as non-transmitters for PERV, possessing the "null" transmission phenotype. The term "null", as coined by (Wood et al, 2004), simply means that despite the presence of PERV-A, PERV-B and PERV-C sequences in the genome of these pigs they lack the ability to infect human or pig cells *in vitro*. This method must be considered the gold standard for determining PERV infectious risk and should be considered compulsory when evaluating new donor herds.

One aspect that can complicate the issue of transmission phenotype is the potential for the transmission status of an animal to change over time. Indeed, data has shown that miniature swine do not maintain their transmission status. For example Wood et al demonstrated that during one 14 month interval, several adolescent miniature swine that were initially capable of infecting pig cells only (non-transmitters) eventually infected human cells thus converting to the transmitter phenotype (Wood et al., 2004). It is unclear if this phenomenon is applicable for other pig breeds, nevertheless any monitoring program of donor SPF herds should include a periodic screening for infectious PERV. Founder animals in New Zealand are tested annually or biennially for PERV infectivity by co-culturing with target cell lines and data has shown that these animals have retained their PERV null phenotype for more than 6 years (Wynyard, 2011).

4.2 PERV expression and RT activity

In addition to studying *in vitro* co-culture infectivity it is recommended that the PERV viral load and RT activity is measured in donor blood plasma. During the characterisation of the

New Zealand SPF herd PERV viral load in donor blood plasma was measured by real-time PCR using a methodology similar to that described by Dieckhoff et al (2009). RT activity that would indicate retroviral activity and therefore the presence of retroviral particles was also measured in the blood of the donors using a C-Type RT kit (Garkavenko, Wynyard, Nathu, Muzina, et al., 2008; Garkavenko, Wynyard, Nathu, Simond, et al., 2008). No evidence of PERV expression or RT activity in pig donors' blood plasma or from stimulated PBMC was found.

4.3 PERV gene dosage (copy number)

Pigs that possess a low number of PERV provirus within their genome will theoretically pose less infectious risk than those with a high copy number. This is because the majority of PERV sequences appear to be either defective or deleted, i.e., they contain only one or two intact retro- viral open reading frames of *gag*, *pol* and *env* (Bosch, Arnauld, & Jestin, 2000; Czauderna, Fischer, Boller, Kurth, & Tonjes, 2000; Herring et al., 2001; Niebert, Rogel-Gaillard, Chardon, & Tonjes, 2002). Consequently PERV proviral copy number is another important characteristic that should be investigated when assessing a donor herd for infectious risk. This data can be obtained using a real-time PCR absolute quantification methodology. If this is not feasible then a laboratory may employ the simpler PCR based limited dilution assay (PLDA). PLDA has been widely used to quantify different target molecules, including human immunodeficiency virus copy number (Rodrigo, Goracke, Rowhanian, & Mullins, 1997). The New Zealand SPF herd has been screened using both methods (Wynyard, 2011; Wynyard, Garkavenko, & Elliott, 2011) for which a high concordance was observed. PERV copy number in NZ SPF pigs varied from 3 to 68 copies per cell with an average copy number of 17.6 and were found to be not statistically different from the NZ landrace breed or more interestingly the Miniature Swine breed that are known to infect human cells *in vitro* (Patience, 1997; Takeuchi, 1998). These techniques provide a sensitive and reliable method to specifically identify animals with low PERV copy number (<10 copies per cell) that are suitable for further selective breeding. Numerous such individual pigs have been identified in the AI pig herd and are currently being bred to reduce PERV infectious risk.

4.4 PERV recombinants

Another important aspect to consider is the ability of PERV-A and PERV-C to recombine as there is evidence that PERV A/C recombinants show higher titres when cultured in human cells *in vitro* (Bartosch et al., 2004; Oldmixon et al., 2002; Wilson, Wong, VanBrocklin, & Federspiel, 2000; Wood et al., 2004). As discussed earlier, using the co-culture infectivity test with human HEK293 and swine St Iowa target cell lines, it was established that primary cells (PBMCs) from NZ donor pigs do not release either xeno- or ecotropic infective viruses (Garkavenko, Wynyard, Nathu, Muzina, et al., 2008; Garkavenko, Wynyard, Nathu, Simond, et al., 2008). To support the lack of transmission from this herd, animals were tested for and found to lack the genomic presence of high titre recombinant PERV A/C. A potential PERV-C locus that may contribute to recombination and the generation of transmissible PERV sequences in miniature swine was also found to be absent. These animals also appear to be transcriptionally inactive for PERV-C as PERV-C RNA could not be detected despite possessing PERV-C proviral sequences.

4.5 PERV infectivity *in vivo*

An assessment of PERV infectious risk can be made at multiple levels beginning with the ability to release virus from the cells of a xenografted organ. Subsequent analysis would need to characterise the virus's ability to cause viremia by revealing productive infection within the recipient cells. Final recognition as a public health hazard would require demonstration of the infectious virus circulating within the patients' bodily fluids. While the ability of PERV to infect human cells *in vitro* is well documented, less is actually known about PERV infectious potential *in vivo* and its capacity to cause disease. To address this question numerous animal models have been investigated. The most common models have been concentrated around the use of non-human primates (NHP) or small animals such as severe combined immunodeficiency (SCID) mice. Unfortunately both models have proven problematic and in the case of SCID mice somewhat contentious. In NHP, conflicting results have been reported as regards the resistance of NHP cells to PERV infection, with some studies reporting non-permissiveness (Martin, Steinhoff, Kiessig, Chikobava, Anssar et al, 1999; Patience et al, 1997; Takeuchi et al, 1998; Wilson et al, 2000) and others suggesting susceptibility (Blusch, Patience, Takeuchi, Templin, Von Der Helm et al, 2000; Specke, Tacke, Boller, Schwendemann & Denner, 2001; Templin, Schroder, Simon, Laaff, Kohl et al, 2000). For mice the situation is more complicated. Originally it was discovered that PERV, produced from pig pancreatic cells and transplanted into SCID mice, could infect mouse tissues *in vivo*. However, the virus produced appeared to be transcriptionally inactive, signifying a non-productive infection (van der Laan, Lockey, Griffeth, Frasier, Wilson et al, 2000). Subsequent analysis revealed that this was not a true infection but rather evidence of pseudotyping involving the collaboration of mouse (endogenous xenotropic MLV) and PERV retroviral elements (Martina, Kurian, Cherqui, Evanoff, Wilson et al, 2005). In terms of overall success, despite several studies demonstrating the transmission of PERV *in vivo* (Argaw, Colon-Moran & Wilson, 2004; Martina, Marcucci, Cherqui, Szabo, Drysdale et al, 2006; Popp, Mann, Milburn, Gibbs, McCullagh et al, 2007), no report has conclusively demonstrated productive infection (Denner, Specke, Karlas, Chodnevskaja, Meyer et al, 2008; Hermida-Prieto, Domenech, Moscoso, Diaz, Ishii et al, 2007; Levy, Argaw, Wilson, Brooks, Sandstrom et al, 2007; Moscoso, Hermida-Prieto, Manez, Lopez-Pelaez, Centeno et al, 2005; Paradis, Langford, Long, Heneine, Sandstrom et al, 1999; Specke, Schuurman, Plesker, Coulibaly, Ozel et al, 2002). In terms of *in vivo* transmission from the AI pig herd no evidence of PERV infection was found in non-human primates following transplantation of islet cells (Garkavenko, Dieckhoff, Wynyard, Denner, Elliott et al, 2008) or in twelve human patients sampled from the New Zealand clinical trial (Wynyard, 2011).

Such a predominance of data against PERV infection *in vivo* begs the question as to whether PERV is of real importance. On the other hand it may just be a case of having not yet found a suitable animal model. It is worth noting that the difficulties associated with PERV *in vivo* infection may also be attributed to the inconsistency of methods used for PERV detection in recipients. Indeed the detection of all PERV subtypes, especially PERVA/C, may not be adequately covered by currently employed PCR and serological methodologies. Establishing quality testing practices therefore becomes vital.

5. Patient follow up and laboratory standards

Approval for clinical trials in xenotransplantation requires comprehensive regulation and approval by government authorities. Crucial to any successful application is demonstration that the methodologies employed to test both donor animals and xenograft recipients are current and accurate. The Molecular Diagnostic Laboratory responsible for testing the New Zealand SPF donor herd and transplant patients employs both serological (ELISA, Late Agglutination Test) and molecular techniques (PCR, real-time PCR) as part of its testing program. However the preferred methodology is a multiplex High Resolution Melting (HRM) real-time PCR similar to that described in (Wynyard, 2011). In this study the superior melting properties of the HRM chemistry enable the simultaneous amplification of sequences for PERV *pol*, Cytochrome Oxidase II (a pig cell marker) and a heterologous internal control in a single multiplexed reaction. This assay has been employed successfully to screen 12 xenograft recipients of porcine islets to exclude PERV infection whilst simultaneously checking for template integrity, PCR inhibition and microchimerism. Research groups expecting to perform xeno-testing must be prepared to show competencies with nucleic acid methodologies preferably with expertise in both veterinary and medical diagnostic fields. For pathogens that lack commercially available tests or where in-house capabilities are insufficient then a network of reference laboratories and collaborators maybe employed to perform the tests instead. All assays should be suitably validated to ensure accuracy, reproducibility, specificity and sensitivity (both analytical and where possible diagnostic) as expected from any medical diagnostic laboratory (American Association of Veterinary Laboratory Diagnosticians, 2010; Raymaekers, Bakkus, Boone, de Rijke, El Housni et al, 2011). It is important that assays for pathogens that are screened in donor animals show equal efficacy when tested from human tissues and validation protocols should account for this. Controls are mandatory and it is recommended that suitable internal controls are incorporated to improve assay reliability (Hoorfar, Malorny, Abdulmawjood, Cook, Wagner et al, 2004). For example in the New Zealand diagnostic laboratory tissues destined for real-time PCR analysis are routinely spiked with a heterologous internal control that can be used to infer nucleic acid integrity and PCR inhibition (Wynyard, 2011; assays in preparation for publication).

To achieve the highest diagnostic standards it is advisable that laboratories expecting to perform xenomicrobiology testing are accredited to international standards. This will facilitate the use of suitable methods and that laboratory staff are trained and competent to perform each assay. Moreover, accreditation ensures that a suitable QA/QC program is put in place to guarantee that results are reliable and can be trusted. The NZ testing laboratory is audited annually and registered with International Accreditation New Zealand (IANZ). Accreditation is maintained to the ISO15189:2007 standard. It is important to note that for the screening of both the herd and recipients that robust protocols for managing positive results are established. This encompasses the confirmatory testing needed to exclude false positives and describes clearly defined communication lines for reporting. Reporting contacts may include the animal facilities, executive management, pig handlers or in the case of positive results for non-endemic pathogens, the involvement of government departments responsible for biosecurity, animal welfare and public health. Full documentation (integral to the accreditation process) is essential for providing traceability when subject to auditing by regulatory bodies.

6. Conclusions

Any xenotransplantation project should consider a comprehensive safety program that includes two key aspects - donor monitoring and patients' follow-up. Initial identification of donor herds suitable for xenotransplantation requires a comprehensive understanding of viral epidemiology within pig populations and an understanding of the relevant viruses as dictated by the geographical area. A clear decision making process is required to exclude animals that carry infectious agents that ultimately requires a risk versus benefit analysis. Upon the selection of suitable pig donor herd a multilevel screening program is required that tests donor material from breeding animals at the herd level through to the final product. Strategies for management of positive animals must be in place to minimize the risk to the donor herd and transplant recipients. PERV remains the central safety consideration in xenotransplantation. It is very important to develop a standard approach towards the characterization of PERV infectious potential within a potential donor herd. Such a benchmark allows for the comparison of PERV characteristics from pig donors of different backgrounds and ensures the selection of techniques and methods that are reliable and practical for the industry. To effectively characterize PERV in source animals requires a rigorous PERV screening program as has been implemented in a New Zealand specific pathogen free (SPF) pig herd. The key elements of this program should consist of: (a) testing for *in vitro* infectivity of both eco- and xenotropic viruses using standard cell culture infectivity methods (Patience, Takeuchi, & Weiss, 1997); (b) measuring reverse transcriptase (RT) activity and PERV viral expression in donors' blood plasma (Dieckhoff et al., 2009; Garkavenko, Wynyard, Nathu, Muzina, et al., 2008; Garkavenko, Wynyard, Nathu, Simond, et al., 2008); (c) measuring the PERV proviral copy number per cell (Wynyard, 2011) and (d) testing for the presence or absence of PERV recombinants and a potential PERV-C loci that may contribute to recombination and the generation of highly transmissible PERV sequences (Garkavenko, Wynyard, Nathu, Muzina, et al., 2008; Garkavenko, Wynyard, Nathu, Simond, et al., 2008). These data provide the basis for a selective pig breeding program with the ultimate goal of enhancing the safety of donors for cell transplantation by minimising PERV infectious risk. It should be evident that patient safety relies heavily upon a robust program of monitoring in transplant recipients. It is expected that laboratory practices meet international standards to ensure technical competence and result validity.

The strategies described in this chapter have been successfully applied in New Zealand and proven crucial towards facilitating clinical trials using porcine islets. It is expected that the same strategies will find broad application outside of New Zealand and provide sufficient guidelines to benefit interested parties looking to enter the xenotransplantation field.

7. References

Alexander, D. J. & Brown, I. H. (2000). Recent zoonoses caused by influenza A viruses. *Revue scientifique et technique*, 19, 97-225.

American Association of Veterinary Laboratory Diagnosticians. (2010). Requirements for an Accredited Veterinary Medical Diagnostic Laboratory. Date of Access: 20 July 2011. Available from: http://www.aavld.org/index.php?option=com_content&view=article&id=18&Itemid=85

Argaw, T.; Colon-Moran, W. & Wilson, C. A. (2004). Limited infection without evidence of replication by porcine endogenous retrovirus in guinea pigs. *Journal of General Virology*, 85(Pt 1), 15-19.

Bartosch, B.; Stefanidis, D.; Myers, R.; Weiss, R.; Patience, C. & Takeuchi, Y. (2004). Evidence and consequence of porcine endogenous retrovirus recombination. *Journal of Virology*, 78(24), 13880-13890.

Blusch, J. H.; Patience, C.; Takeuchi, Y.; Templin, C. C. R.; Von Der Helm, K.; Steinhoff, G. & Martin, U. (2000). Infection of Nonhuman Primate Cells by Pig Endogenous Retrovirus. *Journal of Virology*, 74(16), 7687-7690.

Bogdan, J.; West, K.; Clark, E.; Konoby, C.; Haines, D.; Allan, G.; McNeilly, F.; Meehan, B.; Krakowka, S. & Ellis, J. A. (2001). Association of porcine circovirus 2 with reproductive failure in pigs: A retrospective study. *Canadian Veterinary Journal*, 42(7), 548–550.

Bosch, S.; Arnauld, C. & Jestin, A. (2000). Study of full-length porcine endogenous retrovirus genomes with envelope gene polymorphism in a specific-pathogen-free Large White swine herd. *Journal of Virology*, 74(18), 8575-8581.

Bush, R. M. (2004). Influenza as a model system for studying the cross-species transfer and evolution of the SARS coronavirus. *Philosophical Transactions of the Royal Society B: Biological Sciences*, 359, 1067–1073.

Celera, V. J. & Carasova, P. (2002). First evidence of porcine circovirus type 2 (PCV-2) infection of pigs in theCzech Republic by seminested PCR. *Journal of veterinary medicine B: Infectious diseases and veterinary public health*, 49(3), 155–159.

Czauderna, F.; Fischer, N.; Boller, K.; Kurth, R. & Tonjes, R. R. (2000). Establishment and characterization of molecular clones of porcine endogenous retroviruses replicating on human cells. *Journal of Virology*, 74(9), 4028-4038.

Denner, J. (2008). Is porcine endogenous retrovirus (PERV) transmission still relevant? *Transplantation Proceedings*, 40(2), 587-589.

Denner, J.; Specke, V.; Karlas, A.; Chodnevskaja, I.; Meyer, T.; Moskalenko, V.; Kurth, R. & Ulrichs, K. (2008). No transmission of porcine endogenous retroviruses (PERVs) in a long-term pig to rat xenotransplantation model and no infection of immunosuppressed rats. Annals of Transplantation, 13(1), 20-31.

Dieckhoff, B.; Kessler, B.; Jobst, D.; Kues, W.; Petersen, B.; Pfeifer, A.; Kurth, R.; Niemann, H.; Wolf, E. & Denner, J. (2009). Distribution and expression of porcine endogenous retroviruses in multi-transgenic pigs generated for xenotransplantation. *Xenotransplantation*, 16(2), 64-73.

Dorrschuck, E.; Munk, C. & Tonjes, R. R. (2008). APOBEC3 proteins and porcine endogenous retroviruses. *Transplantation Proceedings*, 40(4), 959-961.

Fiane, A. E.; Mollnes, T. E. & Degre, M. (2000). Pig endogenous retrovirus - a threat to clinical xenotransplantation? *Apmis*, 108(4), 241-250.

Fishman, J. A. (2001a). Infection in Xenostransplantation. *Journal of Cardiac Surgery*, 16(5), 363-373.

Fishman, J. A. (2001b). Prevention of infection in xenotransplantation. In J. L. Platt (Ed.), *Xenotransplantation*. Washington, D.C: ASM Press.

Gao, F.; Bailes, E.; Robertson, D. L.; Chen, Y. L.; Rodenburg, C. M.; Michael, S. F.; Cummins, L. B.; Arthur, L. O.; Peeters, M.; Shaw, G. M.; Sharp, P. M. & Hahn, B. H. (1999).

Origin of HIV-1 in the chimpanzee Pan troglodytes troglodytes. *Nature*, 397(6718), 436-441.

Garkavenko, O.; Croxson, M. C.; Irgang, M.; Karlas, A.; Denner, J. & Elliott, R. B. (2004). Monitoring for presence of potentially xenotic viruses in recipients of pig islet xenotransplantation. *Journal of Clinical Microbiology*, 42(11), 5353-5356.

Garkavenko, O.; Dieckhoff, B.; Wynyard, S.; Denner, J.; Elliott, R. B.; Tan, P. L. & Croxson, M. C. (2008). Absence of Transmission of Potentially Xenotic Viruses in a Prospective Pig to Primate Islet Xenotransplantation Study. *Journal of Medical Virology*, 80, 2046–2052.

Garkavenko, O.; Elliott, R. B. & Croxson, M. C. (2005). Identification of pig circovirus type 2 in New Zealand pigs. *Transplantation Proceedings*, 37(1), 506-509.

Garkavenko, O.; Muzina, M.; Muzina, Z.; Powels, K.; Elliott, R. B. & Croxson, M. C. (2004). Monitoring for potentially xenozoonotic viruses in New Zealand pigs. *Journal of Medical Virology*, 72(2), 338-344.

Garkavenko, O.; Obriadina, A.; Meng, J.; Anderson, D. A.; Benard, H. J.; Schroeder, B. A.; Khudyakov, Y. E.; Fields, H. A. & Croxson, M. C. (2001). Detection and characterisation of swine hepatitis E virus in New Zealand. *Journal of Medical Virology*, 65(3), 525-529.

Garkavenko, O.; Wynyard, S.; Nathu, D.; Muzina, M.; Muzina, Z.; Scobie, L.; Hector, R. D.; Croxson, M. C.; Tan, P. & Elliott, B. R. (2008). Porcine endogenous retrovirus transmission characteristics from a designated pathogen-free herd. *Transplantation Proceedings*, 40(2), 590-593.

Garkavenko, O.; Wynyard, S.; Nathu, D.; Simond, D.; Muzina, M.; Muzina, Z.; Scobie, L.; Hector, R. D.; Croxson, M. C.; Tan, P. & Elliott, B. R. (2008). Porcine Endogenous Retrovirus (PERV) and its Transmission Characteristics: A Study of the New Zealand Designated Pathogen-Free Herd. *Cell Transplantation*, 17(12), 1381-1388.

Hermida-Prieto, M.; Domenech, N.; Moscoso, I.; Diaz, T.; Ishii, J.; Salomon, D. R. & Manez, R. (2007). Lack of cross-species transmission of porcine endogenous retrovirus (PERV) to transplant recipients and abattoir workers in contact with pigs. *Transplantation*, 84(4), 548-550.

Herring, C.; Quinn, G.; Bower, R.; Parsons, N.; Logan, N. A.; Brawley, A.; Elsome, K.; Whittam, A.; Fernandez-Suarez, X. M.; Cunningham, D.; Onions, D.; Langford, G. & Scobie, L. (2001). Mapping full-length porcine endogenous retroviruses in a large white pig. *Journal of Virology*, 75(24), 12252-12265.

Hoorfar, J.; Malorny, B.; Abdulmawjood, A.; Cook, N.; Wagner, M. & Fach, P. (2004). Practical considerations in design of internal amplification controls for diagnostic PCR assays. *Journal of Clinical Microbiology*, 42(5), 1863-1868.

Kim, J.; Chung, H. K.; Jung, T.; Cho, W. S.; Choi, C. & Chae, C. (2002). Postweaning multisystemic wasting syndrome of pigs in Korea: Prevalence, microscopic lesions and coexisting microorganisms. *Journal of Veterinary Medical Science*, 64(1), 57–62.

Kiupel, M.; Stevenson, G. W.; Choi, J.; Latimer, K. S.; Kanitz, C. L. & Mittal, S. K. (2001). Viral replication and lesions in BALB/c mice experimentally inoculated with porcine circovirus isolated from a pig with postweaning multisystemic wasting disease. *Veterinary Pathology*, 38, 74-82.

Labarque, G. G.; Nauwynck, H. J.; Mesu, A. P. & Pesaert, M. B. (2000). Seroprevalence of porcine circovirus types 1 and 2 in the Belgian pig population. *Veterinary Quarterly*, 22(4), 234–236.

Ladekjaer-Mikkelson, A. S.; Nielson, J.; Storgaard, T.; Botner, A.; Allan, G. & McNeilly, F. (2001). Transplacental infection with PCV-2 associated with reproductive failure in a gilt. *Veterinary Record*, 148(24), 759–760.

Levy, M. F.; Argaw, T.; Wilson, C. A.; Brooks, J.; Sandstrom, P.; Merks, H.; Logan, J. & Klintmalm, G. (2007). No evidence of PERV infection in healthcare workers exposed to transgenic porcine liver extracorporeal support. *Xenotransplantation*, 14(4), 309-315.

Martin, U.; Steinhoff, G.; Kiessig, V.; Chikobava, M.; Anssar, M.; Morschheuser, T.; Lapin, B. & Haverich, A. (1999). Porcine endogenous retrovirus is transmitted neither in vivo nor in vitro from porcine endothelial cells to baboons. *Transplantation Proceedings*, 31, 913-914.

Martina, Y.; Kurian, S.; Cherqui, S.; Evanoff, G.; Wilson, C. & Salomon, D. R. (2005). Pseudotyping of Porcine Endogenous Retrovirus by Xenotropic Murine Leukemia Virus in a Pig Islet Xenotransplantation Model. American Journal of Transplantation 5(8), 1837-1847.

Martina, Y.; Marcucci, K. T.; Cherqui, S.; Szabo, A.; Drysdale, T.; Srinivisan, U.; Wilson, C. A.; Patience, C. & Salomon, D. R. (2006). Mice transgenic for a human porcine endogenous retrovirus receptor are susceptible to productive viral infection. *Journal of Virology*, 80(7), 3135-3146.

Moscoso, I.; Hermida-Prieto, M.; Manez, R.; Lopez-Pelaez, E.; Centeno, A.; Diaz, T. M. & Domenech, N. (2005). Lack of cross-species transmission of porcine endogenous retrovirus in pig-to-baboon xenotransplantation with sustained depletion of anti-alpha Gal antibodies. *Transplantation*, 79(7), 777-782.

Mueller, N. J.; Takeuchi, Y.; Mattiuzzo, G. & Scobie, L. (2011). Microbial safety in xenotransplantation. *Current Opinion in Organ Transplantation*, 16(2), 201–206.

Niebert, M.; Rogel-Gaillard, C.; Chardon, P. & Tonjes, R. R. (2002). Characterization of chromosomally assigned replication-competent gamma porcine endogenous retroviruses derived from a large white pig and expression in human cells. *Journal of Virology*, 76(6), 2714-2720.

O'Connor, B.; Gauvreau, H.; West, K.; Bogdan, J.; Ayroud, M.; Clark, E. G.; C Konoby, Allan, G. & Ellis, J. A. (2001). Multiple porcine circovirus 2-associated abortions and reproductive failure in a multisite swine production unit. *Canadian Veterinary Journal* 42, 551–553.

O'Rourke, L. G. (2000). Xenotransplantation. In C. Brown & C. Bolin (Eds.), *Emerging diseases of animals* (pp. 59–84). Washington, DC: ASMPress.

Oldmixon, B. A.; Wood, J. C.; Ericsson, T. A.; Wilson, C. A.; White-Scharf, M. E.; Andersson, G.; Greenstein, J. L.; Schuurman, H. & Patience, C. (2002). Porcine endogenous retrovirus transmission characteristics of an inbred herd of miniature swine. *Journal of Virology*, 76(6), 3045-3048.

Onions, D.; Cooper, D. K. C.; Alexander, T. J. L.; Brown, C.; Claassen, E.; Foweraker, J. E.; Harris, D. L.; Mahy, B. W.; Minor, P. D.; Osterhaus, A. D.; Pastoret, P. P. & Yamanouchi, K. (2000). An approach to the control of disease transmission in pig-to-human xenotransplantation. *Xenotransplantation*, 7(2), 143-155.

Paradis, K.; Langford, G.; Long, Z. F.; Heneine, W; Sandstrom, P.; Switzer, W. M.; Chapman, L. E., Lockey, C., Onions, D. & Otto, E. (1999). Search for cross-species transmission of porcine endogenous retrovirus in patients treated with living pig tissue. *Science*, 285(5431), 1236-1241.

Patience, C.; Takeuchi, Y. & Weiss, R. A. (1997). Infection of human cells by an endogenous retrovirus of pigs. *Nature Medicine*, 3(3), 282-286.

Patience, C.; Wilkinson, D. A. & Weiss, R. A. (1997). Our retroviral heritage. *Trends in Genetics*, 13(3), 116-120.

Popp, S. K.; Mann, D. A.; Milburn, P. J.; Gibbs, A. J.; McCullagh, P. J.; Wilson, J. D.; Tonjes, R. R. & Simeonovic, C. J. (2007). Transient transmission of porcine endogenous retrovirus to fetal lambs after pig islet tissue xenotransplantation. *Immunology and Cell Biology*, 85(3), 238-248.

Raymaekers, M.; Bakkus, M.; Boone, E.; de Rijke, B.; El Housni, H.; Descheemaeker, P.; De Schouwer, P.; Franke, S.; Hillen, F.; Nollet, F.; Soetens, O. & Vankeerberghen, A. Molecular Diagnostics.be working group. (2011). Reflections and proposals to assure quality in molecular diagnostics. *Acta Clinica Belgica*. 66(1), 33-41.

Rodrigo, A. G.; Goracke, P. C.; Rowhanian, K. & Mullins, J. I. (1997). Quantitation of target molecules from polymerase chain reaction-based limiting dilution assays. *Aids Research and Human Retroviruses*, 13(9), 737-742.

Sachs, D. H.; Sykes, M.; Robson, S. C. & Cooper, D. K. C. (2001). Xenotransplantation. *Advances in Immunology*, 79, 129–223.

Sanchez, R. E.; Nauwynck, H. J.; McNeilly, F.; Allan, G. M. & Pensaert, M. B. (2001). Porcine circovirus infection in swine foetuses inoculated at different stages of gestation. *Veterinary Microbiology*, 83(2), 169–176.

Schuurman, H. J. (2009). The International Xenotransplantation Association consensus statement on conditions for undertaking clinical trials of porcine islet products in type 1 diabetes--chapter 2: Source pigs. *Xenotransplantation*, 16(4), 215-222.

Schuurman, H. J. & Pierson, R. N. I. (2008). Progress towards clinical xenotransplantation. *Frontiers in Bioscience*, 13, 204–220.

Scobie, L. & Takeuchi, Y. (2009). Porcine endogenous retrovirus and other viruses in xenotransplantation. *Current Opinion in Organ Transplantation*, 14(2), 175-179.

Specke, V.; Schuurman, H. J.; Plesker, R.; Coulibaly, C.; Ozel, M.; Langford, G.; Kurth, R. & Denner, J. (2002). Virus safety in xenotransplantation: first exploratory in vivo studies in small laboratory animals and non-human primates. Transplant *Immunology*, 9(2-4), 281-288.

Specke, V.; Tacke, S. J.; Boller, K.; Schwendemann, J. & Denner, J. (2001). Porcine endogenous retroviruses: in vitro host range and attempts to establish small animal models. *Journal of General Virology*, 82, 837-844.

Stoye, J. P.; Le Tissier, P.; Takeuchi, Y.; Patience, C. & Weiss, R. A. (1998). Endogenous retroviruses: a potential problem for xenotransplantation? *Annals of the New York Academy of Sciences*, 862, 67-74.

Takeuchi, Y.; Magre, S. & Patience, C. (2005). The potential hazards of xenotransplantation: an overview. *Revue scientifique et technique*, 24(1), 323-334.

Takeuchi, Y.; Patience, C.; Magre, S.; Weiss, R. A.; Banerjee, P. T.; Le Tissier, P. & Stoye, J. P. (1998). Host range and interference studies of three classes of pig endogenous retrovirus. *Journal of Virology*, 72(12), 9986-9991.

Taylor, L. (2008). Xenotransplantation. eMedicine. Retrieved from http://emedicine.medscape.com/article/432418-overview

Templin, C.; Schroder, C.; Simon, A. R.; Laaff, G.; Kohl, J.; Chikobava, M.; Lapin, B.; Steinhoff, G. & Martin, U. (2000). Analysis of potential porcine endogenous retrovirus transmission to baboon in vitro and in vivo. *Transplantation Proceedings*, 32, 1163-1164.

Trujano, M.; Iglesias, G.; Segales, J. & Palacios, J. M. (2001). PCV-2 from emaciated pigs in Mexico. *Veterinary Record*, 148(25), 792.

Tucker, A. W.; McNeilly, F.; Meehan, B.; Galbraith, D.; McArdle, P. D.; Allan, G. & Patience, C. (2003). Methods for the exclusion of circoviruses and gammaherpes viruses from pigs. *Xenotransplantation*, 10, 343–348.

U.S Food and Drug (FDA). (2001, January 23, 2007). PHS Guideline on Infectious Disease Issues in Xenotransplantation. Retrieved December 14, 2007, from http://www.fda.gov/cber/gdlns/xenophs0101.htm.

van der Laan, L. J. W.; Lockey, C.; Griffeth, B. C.; Frasier, F. S.; Wilson, C. A.; Onions, D. E.; Hering, B. J.; Long, Z. F.; Otto, E.; Torbett, B. E. & Salomon, D. R. (2000). Infection by porcine endogenous retrovirus after islet xenotransplantation in SCID mice. *Nature*, 407(6800), 90-94.

Wattrang, E.; McNeilly, F.; Allan, G. M.; Greko, C.; Fossum, C. & Wallgren, P. (2002). Exudative epidermitis and porcine circovirus-2 infection in a Swedish SPF-herd. *Veterinary Microbiology*, 86(4), 281–293.

Weiss, R. A. (2003). Cross-species infections. Curr Top Microbiol Immunol, 278, 47–71.

Wilson, C. A. (2008). Porcine endogenous retroviruses and xenotransplantation. *Cellular and Molecular Life Sciences*, 65(21), 3399-3412.

Wilson, C. A.; Wong, S.; VanBrocklin, M. & Federspiel, M. J. (2000). Extended analysis of the *in vitro* tropism of porcine endogenous retrovirus. *Journal of Virology*, 74(1), 49-56.

Wood, J. C.; Quinn, G.; Suling, K. M.; Oldmixon, B. A.; Van Tine, B. A.; Cina, R.; Arn, S.; Huang, C. A.; Scobie, L.; Onions, D. E.; Sachs, D. H.; Schuurman, H. J.; Fishman, J. A. & Patience, C. (2004). Identification of exogenous forms of human-tropic porcine endogenous retrovirus in miniature Swine. *Journal of Virology*, 78(5), 2494-2501.

Wynyard, S. (2011). PERV genetic characteristics as selective breeding criteria - developing a pig breed suitable for xenotransplantation. MSc Thesis. University of Auckland, Auckland.

Wynyard, S.; Garkavenko, O. & Elliott, R. (2011). Multiplex high resolution melting assay for estimation of Porcine Endogenous Retrovirus (PERV) relative gene dosage in pigs and detection of PERV infection in xenograft recipients. *Journal of Virological Methods*, 175(1), 95-100.

Ye, Y.; Niekrasz, M.; Kosanke, S.; Welsh, R.; Jordan, H. E.; Fox, J. C.; Edwards, W. C.; Maxwell, C. & Cooper, D. K. C. (1994). The pig as a potential organ donor for man - a study of potentially transferable disease from donor pig to recipient man. *Transplantation*, 57(5), 694-703.

7

The Use of Xenotransplantation in Neurodegenerative Diseases: A Way to Go?

Xavier Lévêque[1,2,3,4], Kyle Fink[1,2,3,4,5,6], Julien Rossignol[5,6]
Gary L Dunbar[5,6] and Laurent Lescaudron[1,2,3,4]
[1]Inserm UMR 643, Nantes
[2]ITUN CHU HOTEL DIEU, Nantes
[3]UFR de Médecine, Université de Nantes, Nantes
[4]UFR des Sciences et Techniques, Université de Nantes, Nantes
[5]Field Neurosciences Institute, Saginaw, Michigan
[6]Department of Psychology and Program in Neurosciences, Central Michigan University, Mt Pleasant,
[1,2,3,4]France
[5,6]USA

1. Introduction

One area of therapeutic research for neurodegenerative diseases consists of cell therapy, which was originally envisioned as a way to replace neurons which were lost in the course of the disease. The early, promising results observed following the transplantation of (embryonic/foetal) neuroblasts in both animal models of Huntington's disease (HD) and Parkinson's disease (PD) and, subsequently, into patients, provided the initial impetus to pursue further studies using this approach. Clinical trials were performed on more than 500 Parkinson's patients and functional improvements were observed in the majority of these patients. However, the lack of recovery and/or the development of long-lasting dyskinesias in a number of these patients, as well as the lack of availability of, and ethical concerns for, the use of human embryonic/foetal tissue led to the cessation of most of these clinical trials.

To avoid ethical and logistical problems relative to the use of human embryonic/foetal tissue and in order to improve the effect of the transplantation, it was important to develop an alternative source of transplantable cells, which was the impetus for using embryonic/foetal tissue from non-human animals. The idea of using xenotransplantation began in 17th century with transfusion of pig blood into human patients to treat high fever for exemple (Roux et al., 2007). Since this initial blood transfusion, xenotransplantation has taken great strides to include transplantation of liver, kidney, heart, lung and brain tissues. Initially it was found that if non-human primates were treated with immunosuppressive agents, pig organs could survive and function for several weeks (Cozzi et al, 2003). However, in many cases, the transplanted pig organs were lost within days or weeks, due to rejection by the host immune system or the host died from complications related to the immunosuppressive treatment. Due to the complications of rejection and use of immunosuppressive drugs, interest in xenotransplantation research waned. However, in 2002, groups of researchers in Boston and Pittsburgh successfully cloned pigs, which eventually led to the creation of transgenic pigs with altered genes that produced a decrease in the local (brain parenchyma) immune response (Groth, 2007).

Xenotransplantion of organ tissues and cells circumvents the issues of donor availability which is one of the major limitations of the use of human embryonic/foetal tissue. The use of porcine cells for xenotransplantation is particularly attractive because of the ease of access to the kinds of cells needed via selective breeding. Furthermore, the ability to plan the breeding to coincide with timing of the surgical implant allows for the possibility to manipulate the donor and/or host cells at the appropriate time in order to decrease the risk of immune rejection of the transplant. Embryonic/foetal pig neural tissue appears to be the most viable source for xenografts into human brain because of the relatively large litters of pigs, and because pigs are amenable to genetic modifications (Sayles et al, 2004). Indeed, studies using porcine (foetal) neuroblasts (PFN) have been successfully conducted using rats and in non-human primates.

2. Xenotransplantation in Parkinson's disease

Xenogeneic neural cell transplantation has considerable promise as a therapeutic approach to treating neurodegenerative diseases, such as Parkinson's disease. Parkinson's disease, first described by James Parkinson in 1817, is characterized by a progressive death of dopaminergic neurons in the substantia nigra, pars compacta (SNc; Hornykiewicz, 1966). The neurons from the SNc in the midbrain project to the neostriatum of the forebrain, providing critical dopaminergic innervation to this structure. Neuronal death in the SNc leads to degeneration of the the nigro-striatal pathway, reducing the dopamine content in the striatum to increasingly lower levels as the disease progresses (Albin et al., 1989). The cause of this degeneration is unknown, but there are some surviving neurons, along with the presence of cytoplasmic inclusion bodies containing an accumulation of normal/mutated neurofilaments. When 70-80% of the dopaminergic neurons die, patients begin to exhibit a postural instability, an akinesia, along with resting tremors. Although, levodopa (the precursor of the dopamine able to cross the blood brain barrier), the most commonly used drug therapy for Parkinson's disease patients provides temporary relief of the major symptoms. Its long-term use can lead to problematic side effects, such as dyskinesia. Deep brain stimulation and surgical lesion of the sub-thalamic nucleus have also shown to be effective in treating symptoms in some advanced Parkinson's disease patients. But, again, these treatments are palliative in nature and tend to reduce the symptoms without providing treatments to reduce the neurodegenerative processes of the disease (Sayles et al, 2004). To date, cell replacement therapies provide the most promising approach to directly address the loss of dopamine neurons in the SNc or provide dopaminergic innervations into the striatum via transplanted dopaminegic cells into or near the striatum (Barker, 2002).

As indicated above, the limitations of using human neuroblasts as a cell replacement strategy has led to the exploration of using xenotransplantation strategies, including the use of porcine neuroblasts to restore behavioral functions in animal models of Parkinson's disease. In 1989, Huffaker and colleagues demonstrated porcine neuroblasts, derived from pig foetal ventral mesencephalum at 21 days of gestation, were able to survive 15-20 weeks in a rat model of Parkinson's disease, albeit with supplements of the immunosuppressant, cyclosporine A (Huffaker et al., 1989). Immunological analysis of the transplanted tissue revealed the presence of tyrosine hydroxylase (TH) positive dopaminergic neurons in grafted striatum. In addition, these investigators observed a positive correlation between the extent of motor recovery and the number of TH-positive cells in the graft. These results were confirmed by others (Galpern et al., 1996; Larsson and Widner, 2000). In addition, clinical trials were performed in 12 idiopathic parkinsonian patients who were given unilateral transplants of 12 million cells (Deacon et al., 1997; Fink et al., 2000; Schumacher et al., 2000). Six of these patients received cyclosporine immunosuppression and six received tissue treated with a monoclonal antibody directed against the major histocompatibility complex class I. Ten evaluable Parkinson's disease patients from both immunosuppressive treatment groups which were given the transplants showed an increase in their clinical scores (>19%) at 12 months post-transplantation. However, post-mortem analysis revealed microglial activation and T-lymphocyte infiltration of the graft, even in the patients given the cyclosporine. These results provided encouraging signs that the PCN transplants could reduce the progression of the disease, but new approaches for addressing the immune response to such transplants were needed.

3. Xenotransplantation in Huntington's disease

Huntington's disease (HD) is an autosomal dominant disorder caused by an expanded and unstable CAG trinucleotide repeat that leads to a progressive degeneration of neurons, primarily in the putamen, caudate nucleus, and cerebral cortex (The Huntington's Disease Collaborative Research Group, 1993). The symptoms of Huntington's disease have been described as early as the fourteenth century, when it was also known as Saint Vitus's dance or dancing plague (Tunez et al, 2010). The disease was first described by Charles Waters as a convulsive disorder, but in 1872 George Huntington formally described it for the first time and referred to it as a hereditary chorea (Huntington, 1872). Huntington's disease is characterized by movement abnormalities, cognitive impairments, and emotional disturbances, which eventually culminates in death around 15-20 years after the onset of motor symptoms. Historically, the neuroanatomical changes in the striatum have been the focus of neuropathological and neuroimaging studies, but more recently, the presence of abnormalities throughout the cerebrum, including cortical thinning and decreased white matter volumes, especially in the prefrontal cortex, have gained significant interest (Stout et al, 2007). Although Huntington's disease has a single genetic cause, it has a very complex pathology, with detrimental effects on a wide variety of cellular processes (Southwell et al, 2009). The most striking neuropathological feature of Huntington's disease -affected brains is the progressive atrophy of the caudate and the putamen, accompanied by a secondary enlargement of the lateral ventricles (Roos et al, 1985). While it is known that the mutation of the gene coding for the protein, huntingtin, leads to widespread brain neurodegeneration, with most of the cell loss occurring in the striatum (loss of medium spiny GABAergic neurons) and cerebral cortex (Reiner et al, 1988), neuronal abnormalities are also found in many other brain regions (Conforti et al, 2008), and it has been discovered that the mutant huntingtin protein can cause malfunctioning and physiological alterations by interfering with transcriptional mechanisms (Borovecki et al, 2006). Currently, only symptomatic treatments are available. Pharmacolotherapy is difficult in Huntington's disease, due to the complexity and amount of damage to the brain. Glutamate antagonists, such as riluzole, have gained significant interest as a treatment for the choric movements associated with Huntington's disease, but the mechanism(s) of glutamate antagonists to slow the disease progression is unknown (Rosas et al, 1999). However, studies of neural transplantation in animal models of Huntington's disease have revealed that grafts of ganglionic eminence tissue into the striatum of Huntington's disease animals can integrate into the host tissue and improve motor function (Bjorklund, 2000).

Researchers have also shown that transplants of multipotent stem cells can up-regulate the proliferation and migration of endogenous neural stem cells, as well increase neural differentiation (Hardy et al, 2008), making them viable candidates for Huntington's disease treatment. Human multipotent stromal cells from bone marrow (hMSCs) have been shown to increase proliferation and induce neural differentiation of endogenous neural stem cells when transplanted into a transgenic mouse model of Huntington's disease (Snyder et al, 2010). However, these transplanted cells were not found in the striatum of Huntington's disease animals at 15 days following transplantation, as a result of necrotic or apoptotic processes (Snyder, et al, 2010). Although the rejection of the xenograft was discouraging, the finding that endogenous neurogenesis was upregulated, even after the graft disappeared, suggests that xenotransplanted cells can recruit endogenous cells even in a short period of time (Snyder, et al, 2010).

Use of human embryonic/foetal tissue for transplantation into the brains of Huntington's disease patients has provided encouraging results, although there are still several problems that limit the clinical utility of this approach, including the limited availability and ethical issues surrounding human foetal tissue (Mazurova, 2001). In 2006, a longitudinal study was conducted that revealed that 3 out of 5 Huntington's disease patients, who received intracerebral grafts of human foetal tissue demonstrated improvement and stability for several years following the transplant (Bachloud-Levi et al, 2006). Even at six years following transplantation, the cognitive abilities of these patients remained stable and only a slight deterioration of motor disability was observed (Bachloud-Levi et al, 2006). However, a more recent study has indicated that only 3 out of 7 Huntington's disease patients who received transplantation of human foetal cells had evidence of graft survival and/or integration into the host tissue at 10 years post-transplantation, although this finding may be confounded by the cyclosporine treatment these patients received for the first six months following the transplantation (Cicchetti et al., 2009).

Xenotransplants of human embryonic/foetal tissue into the rat brain has also been used to test the potential efficacy of this approach for treating Huntington's disease. McBride and colleagues found that human foetal tissue, that was harvested at 12 weeks post-conception and grown as neurospheres for 5 days, and then transplanted into rats that were given intrastriatal injections of the neurotoxin, quinolinic-acid (QA; which causes Huntington's disease -like symptoms), conferred significant neuroprotective properties (McBride, et al 2004). The rats that received both intrastriatal injections of QA and transplantations of human ganglionic eminence tissue into the striatum performed significantly better than rats given the QA only on a motor task up to 8 weeks post-surgery (McBride, et al, 2004). It was also shown that rats given both the QA and transplantation of human foetal tissue had greater striatal volumes when compared to rats given only the QA (McBride, et al, 2004). These results suggest that xenotransplantation of embryonic/foetal cells may be a viable treatment for behavioral and anatomical recovery from Huntington's disease.

Xenotransplantation of foetal tissue has also been tried clinically for Huntington's disease. Transplants of porcine neuroblasts (total of 24 million foetal porcine striatal cells) into Huntington's disease patients, in combination of immunosuppression via cyclosporine or treated with a monoclonal antibody directed against the major histocompatibility complex class I (Fink, et al, 2000), proved to be safe, but did not sustain any improvements in symptoms to the contrary of similarly treated Parkinson's disease patients (as reported above). Over a 12-month period following transplantation, the mean total functionality score was not altered by the treatments in the Huntington's disease patients, suggesting that there were no complications from the treatment. However, the transplanted cells were not capable of slowing the natural progression of the disease, as the motor scores of the patients worsened at the same rate as that of patients who did not receive the transplants (Fink et al, 2000). Whether or not parameters of dosing (e.g., number of cells) or other factors (e.g., genetically manipulating the cells to reduce immunoreactivity) may enhance their clinical utility, remains to be determined.

4. Issues with xenotransplantation

Although transplantation of (foetal) neuroblasts have, thus far, proven to be the best cellular source for restorative therapy for neurodegenerative diseases, the ethical concerns and limited availability of these neuroblasts have led to the exploration of alternative approaches, including the use of xenogenic cells, such as porcin neuroblasts. As noted previously, these cells offer a promising alternative, due to the ease of access through breeding, and the ability to plan the breeding and surgery in a timeframe that allows the possibility to treat both the donor and/or the recipient cells prior to transplantation in a way that could limit the amount of immune rejection of the transplant (Cascalho and Platt, 2001). It is also possible to develop knock-out or transgenic pigs that could be used to limit the immunoreactivity of the transplants and/or increase their efficacy to be tolerated by the brain parenchyma (Cozzi and White., 1995). The choice of porcin neuroblasts as desirable for xenotransplantation is validated by the fact that porcine neurons develop neurites with similar morphology to those observed in allotransplantation of human neuroblasts (Armstrong et al., 2002; Deacon et al., 1994; Isacson et al., 1995). Despite its promise as an alternative strategy to human embryonic/foetal cell transplants, the problems of transplant-to-host infection and potential rejection via strong immunoreactions to the transplant looms as one of the most critical limitations of porcin neuroblast xenotransplants. In terms of transplant-to-host infection, the major concern has been the potential of transmitting an endogen virus integrated in pig genome. Although *in vitro* studies have revealed that porcine endogenous retrovirus in some pig cellular lineages is able to infect human cells, the analyses performed in patients with porcine transplant did not reveal any host viral infections (Fink et al., 2000).

The vulnerability of xenographs to rejection due to a strong immunoreaction remains a focus of much of the work in this area. Although the brain is often considered an "immunoprivileged" organ, there is ample evidence to indicate that a strong immune response within the brain can lead to the rejection of grafted cells. A strong infiltration of the graft by activated macrophages/microglial cells, dendritic cells and T-lymphocytes following transplantation of porcine neuroblasts into the striatum of adult rats has been observed (Finsen et al., 1988; Michel et al., 2006; Remy et al., 2001; Wood et al., 1996).

Activation of these cells can lead to the destruction of intracerebral xenografts. In addition, alteration of the T cell repertoire (Barker et al., 2000), and production of cytokines, such as IL-1, TNF-α, INF-γ, IL-2 and RANTES (Regulated upon Activation, Normal T-cell Expressed, and Secreted), at the site graft, favor a role for TH1 T cells in triggering neural cell rejection (Melchior et al., 2005), while recruitment of dendritic cells early after neural xenotransplantation (Michel et al., 2006) raises the possibility of an active role of these "cell-presenting antigens" in priming naive T cells.

This explains why most of the strategies developed to promote long-term survival of xenogeneic neurons in the CNS have preferentially targeted *cellular*-mediated immune response. Delay in cell rejection can be effectively achieved, but all the approaches used to do this, thus far, involve the use of strong systemic immunosuppression, which can produce serious detrimental side-effects. However, the favourable immunological status of the brain and presence of a minimally-compromised blood-brain barrier raise the possibility of utilizing a local immunosuppression approach to circumvent the problem of rejections of xenografts.

5. Reducing the rejection in xenotransplantation

If xenotransplantation is to become a viable alternative to use human embryonic/foetal tissue for treating either Parkinson's disease or Huntington's disease, one of the first concerns that need to be addressed is finding a way to reduce or avoid rejection of these transplants. Systemic treatment with immunosuppressors, like cyclosporine A (which inhibits T-cell-mediated responses), has been shown to increase the survival of xenotransplants, but has deleterious side effects, such as toxicity to the kidneys. Similarly, daily administration of minocycline (which inhibits microglia activation) can prolong the survival of the porcin neuroblast xenotransplant in the rat, but this drug also has unwanted side-effects (Michel-Monigadon et al., 2010).

Alternative strategies to the use of immunosuppressors following xenotransplantion include the genetic manipulation of the transplanted cells and/or co-transplanting these cells with mesenchymal stem cells (MSCs) or neural/progenitor stem cells (NPSCs) that are known for their immunomodulatory properties *in vivo*. One advantage of the pig as a donor is the possibility of genetic engineering of their cells or organs to exhibit immune properties that favor long-term survival in a xenogenic host. Whereas numbers of genetically-engineered pigs have been created for producing specific type of peripheral organs to be used in xenotransplantation that are less prone to rejection by immune- and acute humoral-responses. One example of this is the generation of transgenic pigs that express the human inhibitory molecule CTLA4-Ig under the control of the neuron-specific enolase promoter (Martin et al., 2005). The hCTLA4-Ig is a fusion protein that blocks the CD28-mediated T cell co-stimulatory signal (Linsley et al., 1991) and stimulates the immunosuppressive activities of antigen-presenting cells in Man and non-human primates (Grohmann et al., 2002). Transgenic neurons, isolated from the ventral mesencephalon or the cortex of G28 pig foetus, secrete hCTLA4-Ig, which binds to human CD80, inhibiting the proliferation of human peripheral blood mononuclear cells in xenogeneic mixed lymphocyte reactions *in vitro* (Martin et al., 2005). The hCTLA4-Ig protein is secreted by transgenic neurons following transplantation into the striatum of rats (Martin et al., 2005).

The efficiency of a local expression of hCTLA4-Ig to promote long term survival of neuronal xenotransplant in the brain is currently under investigation using a non-human primate model of Parkinson's disease (Xenome project UE LSHB-CT-2006-037377). In this experimental model, ventral mesencephalic neuroblasts isolated from hCTLA4-Ig transgenic porcine foetus, are implanted into the striatum of macaques, which were previously injected with MPTP, a neurotoxin that selectively induces the degeneration of nigral dopaminergic neurons. As the hCTLA4-Ig transgene is only expressed in differentiated neurons, all the animals were immunosuppressed with a mix of cyclosporin A, mycophenolate sodium, and steroids, following transplantation. A few months before transplantation, the monkeys were also treated with the cocktail of immunosuppressors, in order to prevent the rejection when the xenografts were initially transplanted, which was prior to their ability to express hCTLA4-Ig. After the transplanted cells were capable of expressing hCTLA4-Ig, the immunosuppressor cocktail was discontinued so that the immunosuppressive effects of the hCTLA4-Ig molecule could be assessed. Preliminary observations indicate that recovery of spontaneous locomotion has been observed in all grafted animals at 11 months post-transplantation (American Transplant Congress, 2010, San Diego, USA). In addition, PET scan analysis using ^{18}F-L-DOPA indicates partial restoration of the intrastriatal dopaminergic activity in at least 5 macaques, while histological analyses show the presence of large porcine grafts composed of dopaminergic, serotoninergic and GABAergic neurons in the striatum of clinically-improved animals. These results suggest that systemic immunosuppression may not be necessary and that local immunosuppressors might facilitate long-lasting survival of xenogenic neurons in the brains of MPTP-treated primates.

Co-transplanting immunomodulatory cells, such as some types of mesenchymal stem cells and neural precursor/stem cells with the xenotransplant may also reduce rejection rates. It is worth mentioning here that if human mesenchymal stem cells (Fig. 1A) are able to express some neuronal phenotypes *in vitro* (Fig. 1B), they do not differentiate easily in nerve cells when transplanted into the brain as compared to neural precursor/stem cells.

Mechanisms of the immunosuppressive effects of these two cell types are not well defined, but some cytokines, known for their immunomodulatory properties, are produced by mesenchymal stem cells and neural precursor/stem cells. The low immunogenicity of these mesenchymal stem cells and neural precursor/stem cells have been correlated to transplant survival (Armstrong et al., 2001; Rossignol et al., 2009), and both porcine neural precursor/stem cells (Michel-Monigadon et al., 2011) and human mesenchymal stem cells (Rasmusson et al., 2005) inhibit T-cell response to anti-CD3/CD28 antibodies or allo-antigens in a dose-dependent way. Thus, grafting of such stem cells could provide an interesting local immunosuppressive environment that could improve xenotransplant survival.

Use of porcine neural precursor/stem cells for co-transplantation with porcin neuroblasts may provide a mean of reducing rejection of this type of xenotransplant. Porcine neural precursor/stem cells grafted in adult rat striatum have been shown to survive longer and induce a weaker immune response than rats given porcin neuroblasts transplants only (Armstrong et al., 2001; Michel-Monigadon et al., 2011). Given these immunomodulatory properties of neural precursor/stem cells, their use in co-transplantation may provide for a more conducive environment for xenografts.

Similarly, the use of mesenchymal stem cells as immunomodulators in xenotransplantation paradigms may result in a decrease in rejections of xenografts. It has been shown that mesenchymal stem cells can prevent dendritic cell differentiation (Ramasamy et al., 2007) and induce anergy of B cells (Corcione et al., 2006). When monocytes and macrophages were cultured with human mesenchymal stem cells, there was a noticeable decrease of pro-inflammatory cytokines and an increase of anti-inflammatory cytokines (Aggarwal and Pittenger, 2005; Nemeth et al., 2009; Spaggiari et al., 2009). A large part of the immunosuppressive effect of mesenchymal stem cells is mediated by soluble factors and, according to previous studies on these cells (Uccelli et al., 2008), several molecules, such as IL-10 or transforming growth factor-β (TGF-β), are potential candidates for the induction of immunosuppression.

In addition, when human mesenchymal stem cells were transplanted into the striatum of healthy rats (Rossignol et al, 2009), the results indicated the presence of only a limited amount of T-lymphocyte infiltration at both 21 and 63 days after transplantation of human mesenchymal stem cells, implying that the immune response is not due to a cellular type response, but, rather, corresponds to an inflammatory reaction (see Fig 1 C, D, E and F). Interestingly, the slight infiltration of T αβ-lymphocytes, which was only observed after vehicle injections, suggests that mesenchymal stem cells inhibited/delayed lymphocyte infiltration into the implantation area. Additional results from flow cytometry revealed that human mesenchymal stem cells do not express class II MHC, excluding them as antigen-presenting cells to T CD4+ lymphocytes and human mesenchymal stem cells express class I MHC molecules, which give them the property of avoiding natural-killer (NK) cell responses (Ruggeri L et al., 2001). Mesenchymal stem cells do not express factors of co-stimulation, like CD40L, CD40, and CD86, which are essential for induction an effective response of T lymphocytes (Majumdar et al., 2003). In addition, they decrease the maturation of dendritic cells, which play a key role in the humoral and cellular immune responses (Guinan et al., 1994). It also appears that mesenchymal stem cells, by interfering with the maturation of dendritic cells, induce a tolerance to the transplant and reduce the cellular responses of T cells (Jiang et al., 2005). Recent work in our lab has shown that human mesenchymal stem cells can be found in the implantation site of all animals at 63, 90 and 120 days after implantation (Fig. 1C, G and H), although some microglial activation were observed (Fig. 1 E). As such, our observations suggest that mesenchymal stem cells are able to reduce the local immune response of the brain that occurs after xenotransplantation.

Moreover, immunomodulatory properties of mesenchymal stem cells could be mediated by inducible nitric oxide synthase (iNOS) and heme oxygenase-1 (HO-1), the latter which, when inhibited, has been shown to completely block the immunosuppressive capacity of human mesenchymal stem cells (Chabannes et al., 2007).

Whatever the precise mechanisms for their immunomodulatory properties, neural precursor/stem cells and mesenchymal stem cells have been shown to provide a local brain immunosuppressive environment that favors engraftment and survival in xenogenic tissue. Understanding the mechanisms underlying the suppressive effect of NSPCs and mesenchymal stem cells could provide critical insights for developing new strategies for local immunosuppression.

In addition to their immunosuppressive properties, mesenchymal stem cells have been shown to produce neurotrophic factors, such as BDNF, GDNF, CNTF, and NT-3 (Rossignol et al, 2011, Uccelli et al., 2008), and porcine NSPCs can trigger an intense innervation of the rat striatum by host dopaminergic fibers coming from the substantia nigra after being transplanted into the striatum (Armstrong et al., 2001).

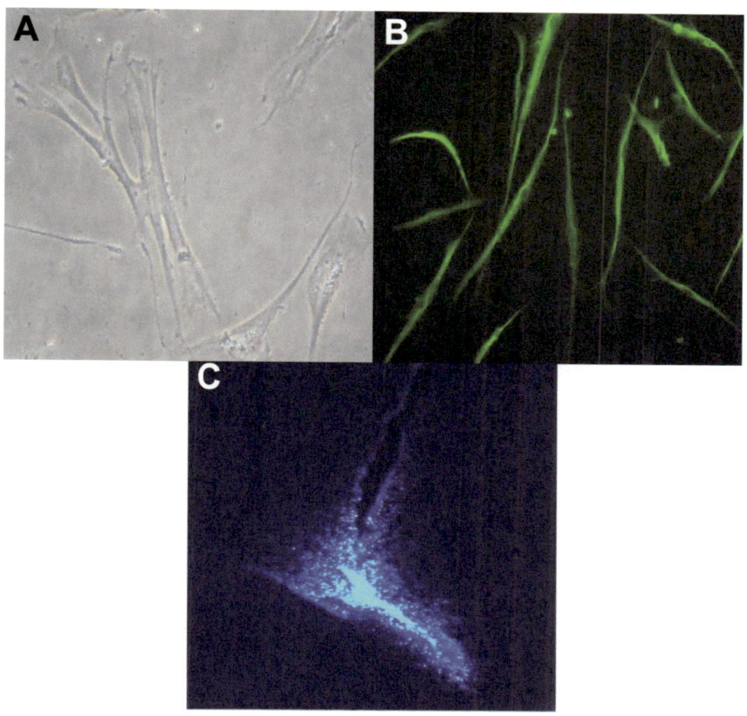

Fig. 1. Morphology of human mesenchymal stem cells (hMSCs) *in vitro* and hMSCs transplantation into the rat striatum.
(A) hMSCs *in vitro* after 4 passages. Note their fibroblast-like morphology. For better transplantation effect, the hMSCs are implanted after 4 passages.
(B) hMSCs labeled with cytoskeleton protein β-Tubulin III. After differentiation using specific culture conditions, hMSCs change shape and are able to express some neuronal markers *in vitro*.
(C) hMSCs labeled in blue with Hoestch 33258 prior to the transplantation are visible inside the striatum after 63 days post-transplantation

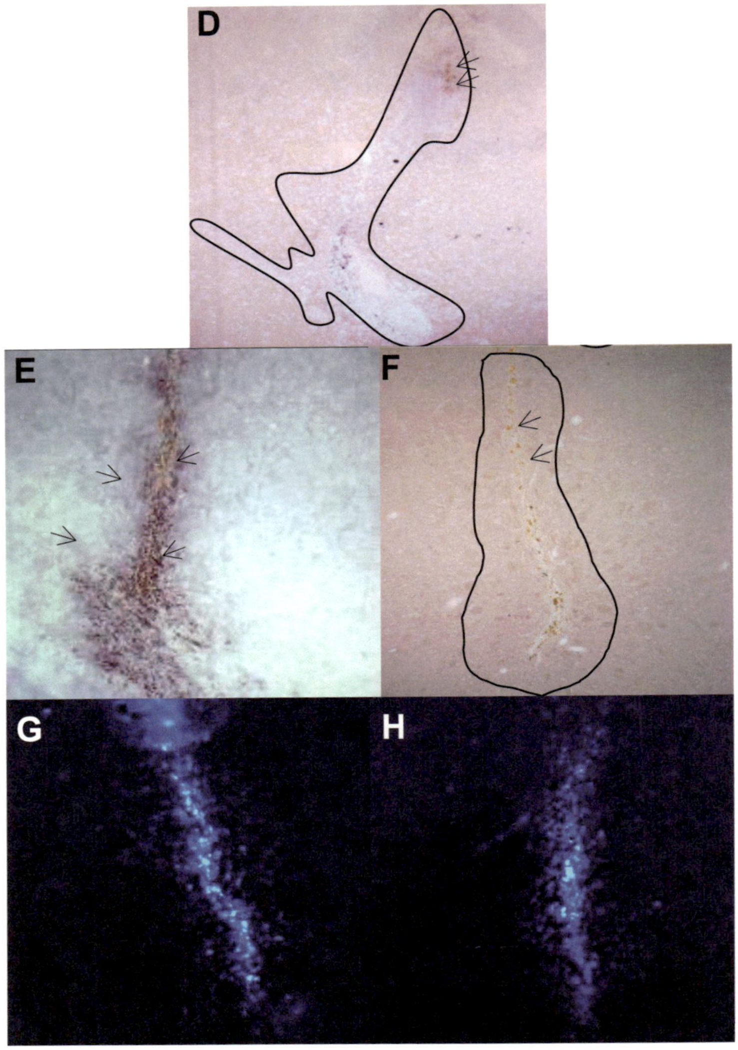

Fig. 1. Continued. (D, E) Same transplant than in (C). Few macrophages/strongly activated microglia (D; arrows) and more activated microglial cells (E; arrows) are present in the vicinity of the transplant labelled with ED1 (D) and OX-42 (E) respectively. However, no sign of transplant rejection was observed.
(F) Sixty three days after the transplantation, very few T-lymphocytes are observed within the implantation site delineated by the dark line (arrows: T-cells stained with R7/3 antibody).
(G, H) hMSCs labeled with Hoestch 33258 prior to the transplantation are visible inside the rat striatum after 90 (G) and 120 (H) days post-transplantation.

The hypoimmunogenic and neurotrophic properties of the mesenchymal stem cells are of great interest for regenerative medicine as they raise the possibility of reconstructing part of the nigro-striatal pathway with xenogenic neuroblasts, in addition to neuroprotective effects on transplanted and/or endogenous neurons. As such, co-grafting mesenchymal stem cells or neural precursor/stem cells with porcine neuroblasts should be considered as a promising approach to increase the effective restorative strategies in the central nervous system and to enhance long term survival of the xenotransplant.

6. Future of the xenotransplantation

Xenotransplantation of foetal tissue for patients who have neurodegenerative diseases offers significant promise. In animal models of PD and HD, the transplantation of embryonic/foetal cells has been shown to be effective in promoting both anatomical and behavioral recovery. However, xenotransplantation of embryonic/foetal tissue typically leads to graft rejection shortly after the transplantation, unless the subject is under constant immunosuppressants. However, for clinical trials in human patients, the use of embryonic/foetal tissue may be limited because of issues of availability (most patients require 2-7 foetuses), tumor formation, and ethical issues. The advent of induced pluripotent stem cells (iPSCs) from allo- or auto-skin fibroblasts may effectively address the issues of availability and ethical concerns and could offer many of the same advantages conferred by the use of embryonic/foetal tissue. In theory, iPSCs should function in ways similar to embryonic cells and foetal tissue following transplantation. However, during the reprogramming phase of iPSCs, known oncogenes such as c-Myc and Klf-4 can be integrated into the genome, potentially compromising the clinical safety and utility of these cells for clinical use. It has also been reported that the reprogramming process associated with iPSCs can lead to genomic mutations, such as expansions and deletions of specific exons, leading to possible genomic instability. In addition, iPSCs are also highly proliferative and have been shown to form tumors when transplanted into immunodeficient mice (Carey et al., 2009). While iPSCs currently hold promise for modelling neurodegenerative diseases, their safety and efficacy needs to be studied extensively *in vivo* before their clinical utility can be adequately assessed. Currently, the therapeutic strategy that appears to best avoid many of the downfalls of human embryonic/foetal tissue, (embryonic stem cells) or iPSCs, is the xenotransplantation of porcine embryonic/foetal cells. As summarized in this chapter, porcine neuroblasts have demonstrated the ability to differentiate into neurons and can avoid rejection if the proper immunomodulation strategy is used. As such, the findings reported in this chapter demonstrate that continued research into ways of improving the efficacy and decreasing the rejection of xenographs warrants further research.

7. Conclusions

The work reviewed in this chapter indicates that xenotransplantation of porcine cells offers several advantages over other therapeutic strategies for treating neurodegenerative diseases, like Parkinson's disease and Huntington's disease. Findings, such as those showing that xenotransplantation of porcine neuroblasts can lead to the differentiation of these cells into neurons and that when the proper immunomodulation strategy is used, these xenotransplants can survive and confer functional improvements in animal models of Parkinson's disease and Huntington's disease (and at least in PD patients), provide significant hope that this therapeutic strategy may be a useful alternative to either transplants of human embryonic/foetal cells.

8. Acknowledgements

This work was supported by La Fondation de France, France Parkinson, CECAP (Comité d'Entente et de Coordination des Associations de Parkinsoniens), L'Association Huntington

France, the RTRS Centaure, La Fondation Progreffe, the Chateaubriand fellowship, the University of Nantes, the Field Neurosciences Institute and the John G. Kulhavi Professorship.

9. References

Aggarwal, S. & Pittenger, M.F. (2005). Human mesenchymal stem cells modulate allogeneic immune cell responses. Blood 105, 1815-1822

Albin, R.L., Young, A.B. & Penney, J.B. (1989). The functional anatomy of basal ganglia disorders. Trends Neurosci 12, 366-375

Armstrong, R.J. et al. (2001). Porcine neural xenografts in the immunocompetent rat: immune response following grafting of expanded neural precursor cells. Neuroscience 106, 201-216

Armstrong, R.J.E. et al. (2002). The potential for circuit reconstruction by expanded neural precursor cells explored through porcine xenografts in a rat model of Parkinson's disease. Exp. Neurol 175, 98-111

Bachloud-Levi, AC. et al. (2006). Effect of fetal neural transplants in patients with Huntington's disease 6 years after surgery: a long-term follow-up study. Lancet Neurology, 5, 303-309

Barker, R.A., Ratcliffe, E., McLaughlin, M., Richards, A. & Dunnett, S.B. (2000). A role for complement in the rejection of porcine ventral mesencephalic xenografts in a rat model of Parkinson's disease. J. Neurosci 20, 3415-3424

Barker, R.A. (2002) Repairing the brain in Parkinson's disease: where next? Mov. Disord 17, 233-241

Bjorklund, A. (2000). Cell replacement strategies for neurodegenerative disorders. Novartis Found Symposium, 231, 7-15

Borovecki, F. et al. Genome-wide expression profiling of human blood reveals biomarkers for Huntington’s disease. PNAS, 102, 11023-11028

Carey, BW. et al. (2009). Reprogramming of murine and human somatic cells using a single plycistronic vector. PNAS, 106, 157-162

Cascalho, M. & Platt, J.L. (2001). The immunological barrier to xenotransplantation. Immunity 14, 437-4468.

Chabannes, D. et al. (2007). A role for heme oxygenase-1 in the immunosuppressive effect of adult rat and human mesenchymal stem cells. Blood 110, 3691-3694

Cicchetti, F. et al. (2009). Neural transplants in patients with Huntington's disease undergo disease-like neuronal degeneration. Proc. Natl. Acad. Sci. U.S.A 106, 12483-12488

Conforti, P. et al. (2008). Blood level of brain-derived neurotrophic factor mRNA is progressively reduced in rodent models of Huntington’s disease: Restoration by the neuroprotective compound CEP-1347. Molecular and Cellular Neuroscience, 39, 1-7

Corcione, A. et al. (2006). Human mesenchymal stem cells modulate B-cell functions. Blood 107, 367-372

Cozzi, E. & White, D.J. (1995). The generation of transgenic pigs as potential organ donors for humans. Nat. Med 1, 964-966

Cozzi, E. et al. (2003). Maintenance triple immunosuppression with cyclosporin A, mycophenolate sodium and steroids allows prolonged survival of primate recipients of hDAF porcine renal xenografts. Xenotransplantation 10, 300-310

Deacon, T.W., Pakzaban, P., Burns, L.H., Dinsmore, J. & Isacson, O. (1994). Cytoarchitectonic development, axon-glia relationships, and long distance axon growth of porcine striatal xenografts in rats. Exp. Neurol 130, 151-167

Deacon, T. et al. (1997). Histological evidence of fetal pig neural cell survival after transplantation into a patient with Parkinson's disease. Nat. Med 3, 350-353

Fink, J.S. et al. (2000). Porcine xenografts in Parkinson's disease and Huntington's disease patients: preliminary results. Cell Transplant 9, 273-278

Finsen, B., Oteruelo, F. & Zimmer, J. (1988). Immunocytochemical characterization of the cellular immune response to intracerebral xenografts of brain tissue. Prog. Brain Res 78, 261-270

Galpern, W.R., Burns, L.H., Deacon, T.W., Dinsmore, J. & Isacson, O. (1996). Xenotransplantation of porcine fetal ventral mesencephalon in a rat model of Parkinson's disease: functional recovery and graft morphology. Exp. Neurol 140, 1-13

Grohmann, U. et al. (2002). CTLA-4-Ig regulates tryptophan catabolism in vivo. Nat. Immunol 3, 1097-1101

Groth, C.G. (2007). Prospects in xenotransplantation: a personal view. Transplant. Proc 39, 685-687

Guinan, EC. et al. (1994). Pivotal role of the B7:CD28 pathwayin transplantation tolerance and tumorimmunity. Blood. 84: 3261–82

Hardy, S.A. Maltman, D.J. & Przyborski, S.A. (2008). Mesenchymal stem cells as mediators of neural differentiation. Current Stem Cell Restorative Threapy, 3, 43-52

Hornykiewicz, O. (1966). Dopamine (3-hydroxytyramine) and brain function. Pharmacol. Rev 18, 925-964

Huffaker, T.K. et al. (1989). Xenografting of fetal pig ventral mesencephalon corrects motor asymmetry in the rat model of Parkinson's disease. Exp Brain Res 77, 329-336

Huntington, G. (1872) On Chorea. Medical Surgical Report, 26, 317-321

Isacson, O. et al. (1995). Transplanted xenogeneic neural cells in neurodegenerative disease models exhibit remarkable axonal target specificity and distinct growth patterns of glial and axonal fibres. Nat. Med 1, 1189-1194

Jiang, XX. et al. (2005). Human mesenchymal stem cells inhibit differentiationand function of monocyte-derived dendritic cells. Blood. 105: 4120–6

Larsson, L.C. & Widner, H. (2000). Neural tissue xenografting. Scand. J. Immunol 52, 249-256

Linsley, P.S. et al. (1991). CTLA-4 is a second receptor for the B cell activation antigen B7. J. Exp. Med 174, 561-569

McBride, J.L. et al. (2004). Human neural stem cell transplants improve motor function in a rat model of Huntington's disease. J Comp Neurology, 475, 211-219

Majumdar, MK. Keane-Moore, M. & Buyaner, D. (2003). Characterization and functionality of cell surface molecules on human mesenchymal stem cells. J Biomed Sci. 10: 228–41

Martin, C. et al. (2005). Transgenic expression of CTLA4-Ig by fetal pig neurons for xenotransplantation. Transgenic Res 14, 373-384

Mazurova, Y. (2001). New therapeutic approaches for the treatment of Huntington's disease. Acta Medica, 44, 119-123

Melchior, B. et al. (2005). Compartmentalization of TCR repertoire alteration during rejection of an intrabrain xenograft. Exp. Neurol 192, 373-383

Michel, D.C. et al. (2006) Dendritic cell recruitment following xenografting of pig fetal mesencephalic cells into the rat brain. Exp. Neurol 202, 76-84

Michel-Monigadon, D. et al. (2010). Minocycline promotes long-term survival of neuronal transplant in the brain by inhibiting late microglial activation and T-cell recruitment. Transplantation 89, 816-823

Michel-Monigadon, D. et al. (2011). Trophic and immunoregulatory properties of neural precursor cells: Benefit for intracerebral transplantation. Exp. Neurol 230, 35-47

Németh, K. et al. (2009). Bone marrow stromal cells attenuate sepsis via prostaglandin E(2)-dependent reprogramming of host macrophages to increase their interleukin-10 production. Nat. Med 15, 42-49

Nemeth, K., Mayer, B. & Mezey, E. (2010). Modulation of bone marrow stromal cell functions in infectious diseases by toll-like receptor ligands. J. Mol. Med 88, 5-10

Ramasamy, R. et al. (2007). Mesenchymal stem cells inhibit dendritic cell differentiation and function by preventing entry into the cell cycle. Transplantation 83, 71-76

Rasmusson, I., Ringdén, O., Sundberg, B. & Le Blanc, K. (2005). Mesenchymal stem cells inhibit lymphocyte proliferation by mitogens and alloantigens by different mechanisms. Exp. Cell Res 305, 33-41

Rémy, S. et al. (2001). Different mechanisms mediate the rejection of porcine neurons and endothelial cells transplanted into the rat brain. Xenotransplantation 8, 136-148

Reiner, A. et al. (1988).Differential loss of striatal projection neurons in Huntington's disease. Proc. Natl. Acad. Sci. U.S.A. 85, 5733-5737

Roos, R. Bots, G. & Hermans, J. (1985) Neuronal distribution in the putamen in Huntington's disease. Journal of Neurological Neurosurgery Psychiatry, 61, 422-425

Rosa, H.D. et al. (1999). Riluzole therapy in Huntington's disease (HD). Movement Disorders, 12, 326-330

Rossignol, J. et al. (2009). Mesenchymal stem cells induce a weak immune response in the rat striatum after allo or xenotransplantation. J. Cell. Mol. Med 13, 2547-2558

Rossignol, J. et al. (2011). Mesenchymal stem cell transplantation and DMEM administration in a 3NP rat model of Huntington's disease: morphological and behavioral outcomes. Behav. Brain Res 217, 369-378

Roux, FA. Sai, P. & Deschamps, JY. (2007). Xenotransfusions, past and present. Xenotransplantation. 14:208-16

Ruggeri, L. et al. (2001). Cellular therapy: exploiting NK cell alloreactivity in transplantation. Curr Opin Hematol. 8: 355–9

Sayles, M., Jain, M. & Barker, R.A. (2004). The cellular repair of the brain in Parkinson's disease--past, present and future. Transpl. Immunol 12, 321-342

Schumacher, J.M. et al. (2000). Transplantation of embryonic porcine mesencephalic tissue in patients with PD. Neurology 54, 1042-1050

Snyder, B.R. et al. (2010). Human multipotent stomal cells (MSCs) increase neurogenesis and decrease atrophy of the striatum in a transgenic mouse model for Huntington's disease. PLoS One, 22

Southwell, A., Ko, J. & Patterson, P. (2009). Intrabody Gene Therapy Ameliorates Motor, Cognitive, and Neuropathological Symptoms in Multiple Mouse Models of Huntington's disease. Neurobiology of Disease, 29, 13589-13602

Spaggiari, G.M.et al. (2009). MSCs inhibit monocyte-derived DC maturation and function by selectively interfering with the generation of immature DCs: central role of MSC-derived prostaglandin E2. Blood 113, 6576-6583.

Stout, J. et al. (2007). Are Cognitive Changes Progressive in Prediagnostic HD? Cognitive Behavioral Neurology, 20, 212-218

Tunez, I. et al. (2010) 3-nitropropionic acid as a tool to study the mechanisms involved in Huntington's disease: Past, Present, and Future. Molecules, 15, 878-916

Uccelli, A., Moretta, L. & Pistoia, V. (2008).Mesenchymal stem cells in health and disease. Nat. Rev. Immunol 8, 726-736

Wood, M.J., Sloan, D.J., Wood, K.J. & Charlton, H.M. (1996). Indefinite survival of neural xenografts induced with anti-CD4 monoclonal antibodies. Neuroscience 70, 775-789

8

Methods and Tools for Detection and Evaluation of the Risks of Porcine Endogenous Retrovirus in Porcine to Human Xenotransplantation

Takele Argaw and Carolyn A. Wilson
Center for Biologics Evaluation and Research,
Food and Drug Administration
USA

1. Introduction

Xenotransplantation has been defined by the Public Health Service as any procedure that involves the transplantation, implantation, or infusion into a human recipient of either (a) live cells, tissues, or organs from a nonhuman animal source, or (b) human body fluids, cells, tissues or organs that have had ex vivo contact with live nonhuman animal cells, tissues or organs (PHS 2001). The promise of xenotransplantation is to provide a replenishable, controlled source of cells, tissues, and organs, in order to alleviate the chronic shortage available for human allotransplantation.

Due to comparable organ size, well defined conditions for breeding and husbandry, and a prolonged co-existence with humans for thousands of years, pigs are considered a relatively safe source for clinical xenotransplantation. However, the finding that the porcine germ line harbors genetic loci encoding porcine endogenous retroviruses (PERV), some of which are infectious for human cells, has hampered clinical development of porcine to human xenotransplantation and resulted in renewed scientific interest in PERVs. FDA's Guidance recommends testing porcine xenotransplantation products, when feasible, by co-culturing with a panel of appropriate indicator cells that could facilitate the amplification of all three receptor classes, PERV A, B, or C (FDA 2001).

PERVs are endogenous retroviruses, and members of the genus gammaretrovirus. Endogenous retroviruses are remnants of ancient viral infections, found in the genomes of most, if not all, mammalian species. Integrated into the chromosomal DNA, they are vertically transferred through inheritance.

In the early 1970s, cultured porcine kidney cell lines were reported to release type C retroviral particles, now known as PERVs (Armstrong, Porterfield et al. 1971). After several studies failed to demonstrate a link to cancer in pigs, progress in studying PERV slowed (reviewed in (Wilson 2008)). In the 1990's, as improved immunosuppressive therapies led to an increase in interest and activity in performing porcine to human xenotransplantation clinical trials, there was a renewal of scientific investigation of PERVs to determine whether they might pose a risk to clinical trial participants. One study demonstrated that the pig cell line PK-15 expressed PERVs that could infect human cells (Patience, Takeuchi et al. 1997) , and our laboratory showed that mitogenic activation of pig primary peripheral blood mononuclear cells was sufficient to release PERVs that were directly infectious for a human cell line in vitro (Wilson, Wong et al. 1998) . These results and those of others who showed transmission of PERV to human cells in vitro (reviewed in (Wilson 2008) framed the debate for the risks of infectious disease transmission in the context of xenotransplantation.

In this chapter we will incorporate research from our own laboratory, combined with a summary of key studies conducted by different investigators. Our own research has been focused in two major areas: 1) to develop tools and methods to facilitate detection and evaluation of the risks of PERV in porcine xenotransplantation products and recipients; and 2) to identify the cellular and viral determinants of human cell infectivity in order to develop strategies to prevent transmission of PERV to recipients of porcine xenotransplantation products. We will provide a review of the published findings of our own lab and those of others describing detection methods and the biological characteristics of porcine endogenous retroviruses (PERV), including their genomic characteristics, and cellular and viral determinants for human cell tropism. The review of the available data will be in the context using living pig cells, tissues, or organs for human xenotransplantation.

2. Investigation of PERV: Paving a way to prevent infection, supporting use of pigs as source animals for xenotransplantation

2.1 Methods and tools development

Availability of sensitive and specific PERV detection methods has been critically necessary to study the biological characteristic of the virus, for screening animals and xenotransplantation products, when feasible, for studying PERV expression and transmission, and for monitoring porcine xenotransplantation clinical trial participants for evidence of PERV transmission from porcine xenotransplantation products. The challenges to development of PERV detection assays include the following issues:

i. Distinguishing between the replication competent form of the virus and replication-defective genomes and transcripts;
ii. Distinguishing between PERV sequences that are the result of microchimerism (surviving pig cells) vs. transmission of PERV to recipient cells;
iii. The potential for genetic recombination between PERVs and other exogenous or endogenous viruses that may compromise the specificity of detection.

2.1.1 Culture assays

Our laboratory had shown that co-culture of pig PBMCs with human embryonic kidney cells (293-HEK) or swine testis cells (ST Iowa cells) provides a sensitive method to detect replicating PERVs released from primary pig cells (Wilson, Wong et al. 1998). Later, we demonstrated that compared to a panel of other cell lines examined, these are the most sensitive cell lines for detection of PERV (Wilson, Wong et al. 2000). Co-culture of pig PBMC with human 293 HEK and pig ST cells provides a sensitive method for screening primary pig cells and tissues for PERV release (Wilson, Wong et al. 1998; Oldmixon, Wood et al. 2002; Wood, Quinn et al. 2004). In addition, pig aortic endothelial cells and human H1080 cell lines were tested as alternative primary source and target cells, respectively, for co-culture assay to screen pigs, though the data from these cells suggest they may not be as sensitive as 293 HEK (Martin, Kiessig et al. 1998).

2.1.2 Pseudotype assay

A primary determinant of retroviral tropism is the surface envelope glycoprotein (SU). By assembling envelope glycoproteins onto the core and genome of a heterologous retrovirus, the tropism of the resulting virus (called a pseudotype) is typically determined by the envelope. Moloney murine leukemia virus (MoMLV), a closely related gammaretrovirus, can be pseudotyped with many different types of retroviruses, including PERV (Takeuchi, Patience et al. 1998) (Wilson, Wong et al. 2000) and can be used as a tool to study viral tropism and the factors that impact the in vitro host range. In order to study the tropism of PERV, we and others have prepared MLV particles pseudotyped by PERV envelopes and used these in a variety of studies (reviewed in (Wilson 2008), and discussed in more detail here, in section 2.2.3). In this assay, pseudotypes are typically generated through the transient transfection of 293T cells with three plasmids: i) one plasmid encoding the retroviral vector genome carrying the packaging signal, deleted for all structural and enzyme coding genes, and in their place, carrying a reporter gene, such as *lacz*, ii) a plasmid expressing the viral core structural and enzymatic proteins, a region of the genome called *gag-pol*, and iii) a plasmid expressing the envelope gene. After 2-3 days, the supernatant from the transfected cells is collected and applied to the target cells to determine the infectivity titer or tropism conferred by the viral envelope (Figure 1). The studies described in section 2.2.3 use pseudotyped viruses to characterize receptor classes, the in vitro host range, and potential species for animal model.

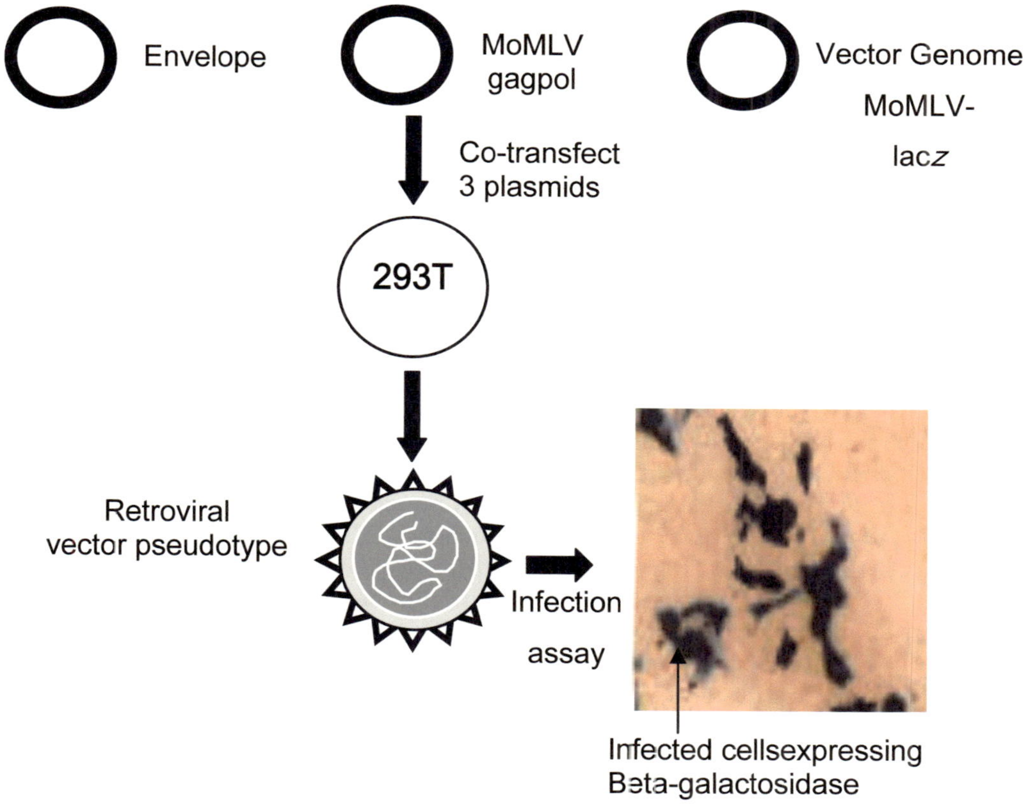

Fig. 1. Typical method used to derive retroviral vector pseudotypes and measure infection properties.

2.1.3 Detection of viral reverse transcriptase activity

Retroviruses carry an RNA-dependent DNA polymerase, also known as reverse transcriptase (RT). Detection of this enzymatic activity provides a unique signature of retroviral infection and therefore, provides a means to monitor the replication of PERV in vitro. The reverse transcriptase (RT) assay is a simple, relatively inexpensive, widely used assay that can detect all retroviruses on the basis of the divalent cation requirement of their RT enzyme, i.e., Mg^{2+} or Mn^{2+}. Basically, in cell or tissue culture when the replication competent viruses exist and continue to expand, the level of the reverse transcriptase activity in the cell culture supernatant increases in correlation to increased virus replication. In the absence of replication, the RT activity may remain low or disappear over time. We and others have used this assay to demonstrate replication of PERVs in a variety of primary cells and established cell lines using an assay based on detecting ^{3}H-TTP incorporation (Wilson, Wong et al. 1998) (Ritzhaupt, Laan et al. 2002). Others have used ELISA-based assays that are available as commercial kits to quantitatively measure RT enzyme (for example, see (Denner, Specke et al. 2008); available from Cavidi AB, Uppsala, Sweden). And a very sensitive measure of reverse transcriptase activity has been developed using PCR-enhanced or PCR-based reverse transcriptase assays (PERT or PBRT; (Irving, Chang et al. 1993; Pyra, Boni et al. 1994), providing a more sensitive and quantitative measure of RT activity, and has also been applied to detecting PERV replication (Patience, Takeuchi et al. 1997; Takefman, Wong et al. 2001).

2.1.4 Quantitative, sensitive detection assays: qPCR and qRT-PCR assays

Sequence analysis of PERV genomes has allowed development of sensitive and specific methods of detection based on PCR amplification. However, the limitation of PCR lies in the inability to differentiate between expression of defective transcripts of the virus and full length replicating virus. However, application of quantitative methods to samples analyzed over multiple time points allows one to determine whether replication is occurring. We have developed quantitative PCR and RT-PCR methods for this purpose (Argaw, Ritzhaupt et al. 2002).

The quantitative PCR (Q-PCR) assay combines sensitivity with specificity and remains a valuable tool to indicate the replication potential of the viruses and for in vivo applications to detect evidence of infection in animals or clinical studies. In this regard, we have developed a real-time quantitative PCR assay based on detection of the PERV *pol* sequence using the *Taq*-Man real-time qPCR technology to quantify PERV RNA or DNA sequences in tissues and cells of human or animal origin (Argaw, Colon-Moran et al. 2004; Levy, Argaw et al. 2007). In this assay, a plasmid construct encoding the PERV-*pol* gene or the in vitro transcribed RNA derived from the plasmid (cRNA) serves as a standard template for amplification of a 178 bp fragment. We have shown that detection of the target sequence is linear over a range from 20 copies to 2 million copies of plasmid DNA and from 100 copies to 1 million copies of the cRNA. This study demonstrated that a real-time (TaqMan-based) quantitative PCR or RT-PCR assay can provide a sensitive, reproducible, and robust method for detecting and quantifying PERV DNA or RNA sequences in samples of human or guinea pig origin spiked with PERV expressing vectors (Argaw, Ritzhaupt et al. 2002) . A similar assay based on SYBR Green I label in combination with primers derived from the PERV *pol* sequence has been used for estimating copy numbers of PERV integrated in the host genome (Bellier, Dalba et al. 2006) .

It is noteworthy that quantitative real-time reverse transcriptase polymerase chain reaction (qRT-PCR) assays have higher specificity and could differentiate between the defective transcripts and the full length proviruses by measuring the level of virus expression at different time points. In this regard, the International Xenotransplantation Association in 2009 recommended that qRT-PCR can be used to assess expression levels of human-tropic PERVs in different pig breeds and source animals (Denner, Schuurman et al. 2009).

When using PCR-based methods to study PERV in animals or clinical trial participants that are exposed to living pig cells rather than cell-free virus, it is important to also incorporate a method to distinguish microchimerism from infection. In other words, survival of pig cells that carry many copies of PERV may confound interpretation of a PCR positive result. Therefore, incorporation of analysis for both PERV-specific PCR and for DNA sequences from pig-specific genes that are highly repetitive, such as mitochondrial or centromeric sequences, is necessary to interpret assays based on detection of PERV DNA by PCR (Switzer, Shanmugam et al. 1999; Paradis, Langford et al. 1999; Blusch, Roos et al. 2000).

2.1.5 Immunoassay

An additional method that is useful to monitor for evidence of transmission in vivo in animal models or human clinical trials, is the use of assays to detect anti-PERV immune responses. Immunologic assays provide the advantage of a rapid assay and one that does not require *a priori* knowledge of the site of viral replication in vivo. However, it does not distinguish between development of an immune response due to viral infection and an immune response due to transplanted pig cells expressing viral proteins. A further caveat to consider is the immuno-suppressive regimens applied in many xenotransplantation clinical protocols and the impact the iatrogenic immunosuppression may have on development of an anti-PERV immune response.

Methods to detect an anti-PERV immune response include antibody detection assays such as Western Blot and enzyme-linked immunosorbent assay (ELISA), functional antibody assays such as lymphocyte fusion inhibition and virus neutralization, and assays of cellular immunity such as detection of PERV-specific cytotoxic T-lymphocyte (CTL) activity and lymphocyte proliferation.

Paradis and coworkers used immunological tests to obtain indirect evidence of PERV infection in 160 patients who had been therapeutically treated with living tissues of pigs. In this study, recombinant protein of PERV-B p30 and purified whole virus, isolated from PERV-infected 293 HEK, were used as antigens to screen for anti-PERV antibodies in serum (Paradis, Langford et al. 1999). Similarly, Matthews and coworkers have used Western blotting for the detection of PERV antibodies in xenotransplantation patients (Matthews, Brown et al. 1999). However, the results and interpretation of data from these studies had the inherent problem of lacking a positive control, as no known human sera exist with anti-PERV antibodies, even amongst the patients who have been exposed to pig tissues. To compensate for no known human positive sera, cross-reactive antibodies developed against simian sarcoma-associated virus (SSAV) and other related retroviruses have been used as indirect controls in assays used to detect PERV antibodies by western blot analysis

(Matthews, Brown et al. 1999). We have also used the anti-SSAV antibodies as a control when detecting anti-PERV p30 antibodies in guinea pigs exposed to either cell-free or cell-associated viruses (Argaw, Colon-Moran et al. 2004) .

In addition to assays used to detect antibody, investigators have also developed PERV-specific antibodies for use in antigen detection assays, as well as to identify neutralizing epitopes. The transmembrane (TM) domain of the PERV envelope was used to derive a goat antiserum that is both neutralizing and can be used for immunoassays such as Western blot and ELISA assays (Fiebig, Stephan et al. 2003). Additional studies have reported development of rabbit-based PERV nucleocapsid anti-serum that can be used for Western blot and immunohistochemistry analysis (Krach, Fischer et al. 2000) . Antisera generated to peptides from the capsid protein (p30) or the surface or TM of PERV envelope class B (SU, gp70(B)) showed functionality in several immunological assays, such as immunoblots, immunofluorescence, and immunogold staining used to detect PERV antigens in biological materials (Fischer, Krach et al. 2003) . Anti-sera raised in different animal species (guinea pigs, sheep, and rabbits) directed against PERV antigens were also evaluated for their use in different immunologic assays for PERV antigen detection (Galbraith, Kelly et al. 2000). A monoclonal antibody specific to the PERV *gag* protien was shown useful for detecting infection (Chiang, Chang et al. 2005) . Recently, a monoclonal antibody directed against the PERV-B envelope protein detected a specific peptide sequence in the proline rich region of SU as an epitope for PERV infection (Nakaya, Hoshino et al. 2011) . These monoclonal antibodies may prove useful for screening for PERV antigen, although to date no xenotransplantation studies have used the antibody on porcine or human xenotransplant recipient samples.

2.1.6 Animal models

While PERV infects and replicates in human cells in vitro, the risk to human recipients of xenotransplantaion products is still unknown. However, the observation that the PERV DNA provirus integration pattern in human cells is observed to be similar to murine leukemia viruses, namely a slight bias towards integration in transcriptionally active genes (Moalic, Blanchard et al. 2006), suggests that from a mechanistic point of view, PERV may be tumorigenic in human cells. Ideally, the best way to test whether PERV is tumorigenic through insertional mutagenesis would be to have a permissive animal model. Unfortunately, in spite of intense efforts by multiple investigators, including our own lab, an animal model of PERV infection, replication, and pathogenesis has yet to be proven, although it would provide an invaluable tool to assess PERV-associated pathology, and evaluate potential prophylactic, therapeutic, or diagnostic medical products.

Initial attempts to identify a permissive animal model for PERV were focused on rodents. Based on unpublished data presented at a public advisory committee meeting of the FDA Subcommittee on Xenotransplantation (13 January, 2000 agenda and transcripts available at: http:// www.fda.gov/cber/advisory/ctgt/ctgtmain.htm), we examined whether guinea pigs would provide a permissive animal model for PERV replication. In an effort to develop a mitotically active organ compartment that might be more permissive for viral infection, we induced the following changes in guinea pigs and then exposed them to cell-associated or cell-free PERVs: i) liver damage by hepatotoxic chemicals to stimulate proliferation of cells permissive to retroviral vectors; ii) initial immunization of the animals with PERV to establish virus-specific antibodies that may enhance infectivity as manifested by other viruses (Olsen 1993; Morens 1994; Yin, Lynch et al. 1999). Despite these measures, we could not detect evidence of replication following exposure of the animals to cell-free or cell-associated PERVs (Argaw, Colon-Moran et al. 2004). Similar results were observed with rats or guinea pigs after PERV was inoculated by either intramuscular or intra-peritoneal routes (Specke, Tacke et al. 2001). No evidence of infection, including lack of detection of anti-PERV antibodies, was shown in immunosuppressed rats transplanted with pig islets (Denner, Specke et al. 2008).

An additional effort to create a permissive small animal model was to introduce the human cDNA expressing the PERV-A receptor, since it was known that the murine ortholog of the PERV-A receptor is reported to be non-functional (Ericsson, Takeuchi et al. 2003) . Exploiting this information, Martina and coworkers, in collaboration with our laboratory, introduced the HuPAR2 cDNA into the germline of mice and generated Hu-PAR2 transgenic mice (Martina, Marcucci et al. 2006). Then the transgenic mice were exposed to PERV, and subsequently qRT-PCR and immunological tests were used to assess viral replication status. Increasingly higher copy numbers of PERV RNA and DNA were detected over the first 2 month period of analysis, although a subsequent decrease in PERV RNA and DNA was observed after 3 months that correlated with detection of neutralizing anti-PERV antibodies (Martina, Marcucci et al. 2006). While not fully explored, the HuPAR-2 transgenic mouse model may provide one model to further study the nature of PERV infection from the perspective of pathogenicity, tissue tropism, and humoral and cellular immunity.

NOD SCID mice transplanted under the kidney capsule with pig pancreatic islets were also evaluated for suitability as a permissive animal model for PERV replication. These studies provided evidence of active viral expression in several tissue compartments suggesting viral transmission (Laan, Lockey et al. 2000) (Deng, Tuch et al. 2000). However, interpretation of these studies changed when a later investigation also performed in immunodeficient NOD/SCID transgenic mice that were transplanted with porcine and human lymphohematopoietic tissues showed evidence of transmission of PERV to the transplanted human cells. The investigators demonstrated that the appearance of PERV positive human cells was most likely due to pseudotyping of PERV C by xenotropic murine leukemia virus, rather than authentic infection by human-tropic PERV (Yang, Wood et al. 2004),. These observations were later confirmed by in vitro studies performed by Martina, et al (Martina, Kurian et al. 2005).

Non-human primates (NHP) were thought by many to provide a good species to evaluate PERV transmission as well as xenotransplant survival by virtue of their phylogenetic closeness to humans, and the use of NHP for evaluation of the effectiveness of porcine xenotransplantation products used in combination with various immunosuppressive therapies to prolong survival in various disease models. Our laboratory demonstrated that NHP cells representing primary and established cell lines from Rhesus, African Green Monkey (AGM) and baboon species were poorly infected, if at all, and that replication is restricted (Ritzhaupt, Laan et al. 2002). These findings were confirmed and extended in a recent study that showed that the ortholog for the PERV-A receptor in rhesus macaque and baboon is non-functional. Similarly, in vivo studies have not found evidence for PERV transmission in NHP transplanted with porcine xenotransplantation products, even when using potent immunosuppression treatments (Moscoso, Hermida-Prieto et al. 2005; Specke,

Plesker et al. 2009). Together, these findings reinforce the conclusion that NHP are not a permissive model for studying the risks of PERV exposure to porcine xenotransplantation recipients.

Studies performed in other species, such as dogs and lambs, have also not shown active viral replication (Edamura, Nasu et al. 2004) (Popp, Mann et al. 2007), leaving the field without a suitable animal model to evaluate the potential for pathogenesis or to provide a means to assess interventions to prevent or treat PERV.

2.2. Genetics and biology of PERV in the context of xenotransplantation

2.2.1 Genome and evolution

Three receptor classes for PERVs have been defined through a combination of sequence alignment and functional receptor studies: PERV A, B and C (Takeuchi, Patience et al. 1998) (Le Tissier, Stoye et al. 1997) (Akiyoshi, Denaro et al. 1998). Analysis of the nucleotide sequence of PERV showed a high nucleotide sequence identity to other gammaretroviral genomes, especially, murine leukemia virus (MLV) and the gibbon ape leukemia virus (GALV), sharing up to 66% identity in the envelope sequence (Le Tissier, Stoye et al. 1997) , and even higher nucleotide identity in the remaining genomic regions, *gag* and *pol* (Akiyoshi, Denaro et al. 1998).

Southern blot and additional genomic analyses have indicated variation in the number, distribution within the genome, and presence of full-length replication-competent genomes, with estimates varying from as low as 3 to as high as 200 copies per genome, depending on the breed and the study (Akiyoshi, Denaro et al. 1998) (Le Tissier, Stoye et al. 1997) (Bosch, Arnauld et al. 2000) (Herring, Quinn et al. 2001) (Rogel-Gaillard, Bourgeaux et al. 1999) (Lee, Webb et al. 2002) (Edamura, Nasu et al. 2004) (Li, Ping et al. 2004) (Garkavenko, Wynyard et al. 2008).

In addition to the known gammaretroviral form of PERV, studies have also identified endogenous sequences in the pig genome representative of the betaretroviral genus (Ericsson, Oldmixon et al. 2001) (Patience, Switzer et al. 2001). Analysis of existing members of the subfamily Suidae and related families suggested that the gammaretroviral sequences representing PERV entered into the subfamily Suidae approximately 3.5 million years ago (Patience, Switzer et al. 2001) (Niebert and Tonjes 2003). The two human tropic envelopes, PERV A and PERV B, have been proposed in one study to predate the pig tropic PERV-C envelope found in members of the genus *Sus* that diverged approximately 1.5 million years ago (Niebert and Tonjes 2005) .

2.2.2 Expression and infectivity of PERV

It has been speculated that there might be tissue- or breed-dependent expression of PERV that might qualify some pig tissues or breeds to be relatively safe for human xenotransplantation. Indeed, the remnants of porcine endogenous retroviruses in genomes of modern-day pigs differ between different breeds of pigs in composition, expression and ability to encode infectious virus. The levels of PERV expression were compared in a large panel of tissues originating from both specific-pathogen free (SPF) and conventional pigs. For all SPF tissues tested, *gag, pol, env*-A, -B and -C mRNA levels were the same range or slightly higher than the corresponding tissues of the conventional pigs. Variation of expression of proviruses was also observed between tissues, with the lowest mRNA levels observed in the pancreas and the highest in the kidney (Clemenceau, Lalain et al. 1999). In other efforts elucidating in vivo expression of PERV, a transmission electron microscopy investigation done on transgenic pigs that express human decay accelerating factor, showed no evidence of active virus release despite the detection of viral mRNA in a variety of tissues analyzed. However, detection of reverse transcriptase activity in pig sera screened in this study, suggested the release of virions into the blood stream (Langford, Galbraith et al. 2001). In a more recent study using semi-quantitative duplex RT-PCR, analysis of gag expression was measured for a variety of tissues in twenty Duroc pigs of different ages, ranging from 10-110 days. While the measurements were not precisely quantitative, the results suggested a trend of highest gene expression in liver and lowest in heart, with some trends of age-dependent gene expression levels, although this varied by organ tested and differences were not great (Moon, Kim et al. 2009).

In addition to in vivo based assessment of PERV expression, several in vitro studies have been conducted to analyze the expression and infectious potential of PERV from various cells and tissues of pigs. Replicating PERV particles have been shown to be released in vitro by cultured primary pig blood vessel epithelial cells (Martin, Kiessig et al. 1998), the pig kidney cell line PK-15 (Patience, Takeuchi et al. 1997) and primary pig peripheral blood mononuclear cells (PBMC) (Wilson, Wong et al. 1998) . We also isolated infectious PERV-C from porcine plasma, as well as pig plasma-derived factor VIII, suggesting that in vivo, blood or endothelium constitutively express PERV (Takefman, Wong et al. 2001). We also could culture PERV-C from freshly isolated pig bone marrow cells by co-culture with pig ST cells (McIntyre, Kannan et al. 2003).

For retroviruses, the long terminal repeat (LTR) carries an enhancer, termed U3 that influences transcriptional activity. Therefore, several studies have evaluated the influence of variant sequences in the U3 region on the level of gene expression for PERV. While our own study did not show significant differences in expression in different cell lines tested for LTRs derived from PERV-A, -B, or –C, we did see a slightly lower level of expression with a chimeric LTR called PERV-NIH and all LTRs tested showed lower expression levels in ST-IOWA pig cells compared to other cell lines examined (Wilson, Laeeq et al. 2003). In other studies, it has been shown that the level of PERV expression in permissive cells is associated with the copy number of a 39 base pair (bp) repeat in the PERV LTR U3 region (Scheef, Fischer et al. 2001). A more thorough study of the LTR structures from kidney of NIH mini-pigs has shown that there are four different elements and that one was associated with the highest level of transcriptional activity. The investigators went on to show that the transcriptional activity could be down-regulated in the presence of a methyltransferase suggesting that transcriptional activity is modulated by DNA methylation (Park, Huh et al. 2010) – a mechanism known to also inhibit gene expression of murine leukemia viruses (for examples, see (Jaenisch 1982) (Stewart, Stuhlman et al. 1982)).

In general, it is likely that only a few of the loci present in the pig genome express full-length replication-competent PERV. However, the polymorphic nature of the integrated endogenous viruses makes it difficult, if not impossible, to identify a breed of "PERV-free" pig. The pig genome sequence project currently running (Archibald, Bolund et al. 2010) and genetic knockout technology may provide more information to guide cloning and breeding of pigs with minimal PERV expression as source animals for clinical xenotransplantation.

2.2.3 Factors impacting human cell tropism of PERV

As described previously, the replication competent PERVs that have been identified to date have been classified into one of three receptor classes, referred to as PERV-A, -B, or –C, based on receptor-specificity properties. As shown in Table 1, both PERV-A and PERV-B are able to infect human cells, but use distinct receptors. Two homologous human cDNAs have been identified and shown to function as the receptor for PERV-A, human PERV-A receptors 1 and 2 (HuPAR-1 and -2) (Ericsson, Takeuchi et al. 2003), but neither of these receptors function as a receptor for PERV-B. The PERV-B receptor remains unknown. PERV-C has a more restricted host range, only able to infect pig cells, and its receptor is also unknown. Interestingly, naturally occurring recombinants between PERV-A and PERV-C have been shown to have increased infectivity titer for human cells compared to the prototype PERV-A (Harrison, Takeuchi et al. 2004).

PERV Envelope	Pig (ST-IOWA)	Human (293)	Rabbit (SIRC) expressing HuPAR-2*
PERV-A	+	+	+
PERV-B	+	+	-
PERV-C	+	-	-

*(Ericsson, Oldmixon et al. 2001)

Table 1. Infection properties of PERV receptor classes

Several studies have analyzed the structure of the HuPAR receptors to identify the functional determinants that allow PERV-A infection. Mattiuzzi and coworkers used the murine ortholog and showed that a single amino acid residue at position 109 in the putative extracellular loop was responsible for the inability of the murine receptor to support PERV-A infection (Mattiuzzo, Matouskova et al. 2007). A later study by Marcucci, et al, showed that there is a 10-fold difference in infectivity titer when PERV-A pseudotypes infect cells expressing HuPAR-1 vs. HuPAR-2. This quantitative difference was exploited to further map the regions within HuPAR-2 that confer this 10-fold increase in infectivity titer. While these studies were unable to define a single residue or group of residues, her results pointed to an additional role of the region encompassing amino acids 152-285 in impacting the efficiency of the receptor to mediate PERV-A entry (Marcucci, Argaw et al. 2009). Interestingly, these studies and others have shown that species-specific polymorphisms of the PERV-A receptors have given rise to PERV-A infection-resistant phenotypes for different reasons. For example, as described above, the murine ortholog is non-functional due to a single amino acid difference, and this observation of a single amino acid change impacting function has been observed for the PAR-1 homolog in rhesus macaque, cynomolgus macaque, and baboon (all have serine at amino acid residue 109) (Mattiuzzo and Takeuchi 2010). However, the rat PAR allows PERV-A infection when expressed in non-permissive cell lines, although rat cells do not support PERV-A entry. Mattiuzzo, and coworkers, have data suggesting that the endogenous receptor expression in rat cells is too low to allow PERV-A infection (Mattiuzzo, Matouskova et al. 2007).

The normal cellular function for the human PERV-A receptors is somewhat controversial, in that there are two independent reports of screens that identified very different functions for the PERV-A receptor: a CNS-specific receptor for gamma-hydroxybutyrate, hypothesized to be a G-protein-linked receptor (Andriamampandry, Taleb et al. 2007; 2008); and a riboflavin transporter, termed RFT1 (Yonezawa, Masuda et al. 2008). While neither study has been followed with additional publications to confirm or deny each of the reported claims, the latter report makes more sense, when the tissue-specific pattern of PERV-A receptor expression and identified gammaretroviral receptors, in general, are taken into account: 1) The PERV-A receptor mRNA has been shown to be widely expressed (Ericsson, Takeuchi et al. 2003), similar to what has been shown for RFT1 (Yonezawa, Masuda et al. 2008); 2) Both RFT1 and PAR have been predicted to have ten transmembrane domains; 3) All receptors identified to date for gammaretroviruses are Class 2A carrier-type facilitator transporters (Hein, Prassolov et al. 2003).

While detailed understanding of the cellular factors required for human cell infection is critical, an equally important area of study is that of cellular restriction factors. Only in relatively recent years, primarily driven by HIV research, have cellular restriction factors been identified (Neil and Bieniasz 2009). While a number of restriction factors have been identified that restrict HIV or other retroviruses from infecting certain cell types, not all necessarily have been shown to also restrict PERV infection. For example, TRIM5α molecules have been shown to restrict a variety of lentiviruses and some gammaretroviruses in a species-specific manner. However, none of the primate or non-primate-derived TRIM-5α, including those from human, African green monkey, squirrel monkey, rhesus macaque, cattle, and rabbit, inhibited infection by PERV-A or a naturally occurring recombinant, PERV-A/C (Wood, Webb et al. 2009). In contrast, there is limited evidence to suggest that two other known restriction factors may have species-specific restriction of PERV replication. Mattiuzzo, et al, demonstrated that the level of processed *gag* in the cell lysate and supernatant was inversely correlated with expression levels of the late-acting restriction factor called tetherin (Mattiuzzo and Takeuchi 2010). These observations suggest that certain non-human primate cells may restrict PERV replication due to a late stage defect in *gag* processing and virus particle release – observations that confirm and extend observations from our earlier study on restriction to PERV replication in non-human primate cells (Ritzhaupt, Laan et al. 2002). Another restriction factor identified initially in studies with HIV is called APOBEC – it is packaged into viral particles and inhibits viral replication by editing cytosine residues through its deaminase activity (reviewed in (Goila-Gaur and Strebel 2008)). Recently, the porcine APOBEC proteins were identified and analyzed for their ability to restrict PERV replication and it was shown that they were packaged into the PERV virions and edited certain cytosine residues, suggesting that this may be a mechanism by which porcine cells restrict this endogenous retrovirus (Dorrschuck, Fischer et al. 2011). Although some have hypothesized that human APOBEC may restrict PERV replication to account for the observed lack of transmission in human xenotransplantation clinical trial participants (see section 2.2.4), a detailed study to determine whether human APOBEC might also restrict PERV has not been performed, to date.

In addition to trying to understand the cellular determinants of human cell tropism of PERV, efforts have also been directed towards looking at the viral determinants of human cell infection. In general, the primary determinant of cell tropism is the viral envelope. Our laboratory has used a variety of approaches to identify the region of the PERV-A envelope required for human cell infection: binding assays, pseudotype infectivity assays, and generation of recombinant and site-directed variants of envelope to assess structure-function relationships. Using a fusion protein based on the rabbit immunoglobulin heavy chain, we showed several years ago that PERV envelope binding requires a region beyond the prototypical receptor binding domain (RBD) for gammaretroviruses. As shown in Figure 2, the RBD that we mapped using this approach encompassed not just the variable regions A and B (VRA and VRB) as has been shown for other related viruses, but also requires the proline-rich region (PRR) (Gemeniano, Mpanju et al. 2006). Using the pseudotype assay described in section 2.1.5, we and others have tried to identify more precisely the regions of the envelope required for human cell infection. Harrison et al used a naturally occurring recombinant of PERV-A and PERV-C with high titer on human cells compared to parental PERV-A and showed two regions that correlated with increased infection on human cells: amino acid residue 140 that lies between VRA and VRB and additional sequences within the PRR (Harrison, Takeuchi et al. 2004). Our laboratory has also shown that sequences within the C-terminal region of the SU influence human cell infectivity (Gemeniano, Mpanju et al. 2006; Argaw, Figueroa et al. 2008).

We have also shown that PERV-C RBD can bind human cells specifically, in a dose-dependent manner (Gemeniano, Mpanju et al. 2006). More recently, we demonstrated that relatively few amino acid changes in the PERV-C envelope can allow infection of human cells (Argaw, Figueroa et al. 2008). Together, these results suggest that human cells may carry PERV-C receptors that are non-functional for wild-type PERV-C infection, but allow binding, and that just a few amino acid changes within the PERV-C envelope allow entry. Our lab has further shown that the molecule that binds PERV-C and allows mutant PERV-C to infect human cells is distinct from the human PERV-A receptor (Gemeniano, Mpanju et al. 2006; Argaw, Figueroa et al. 2008). These observations suggest that with long-term survival of porcine xenotransplantation products that do not carry PERV-A or other human-tropic forms of PERV naturally, that over time, mutant PERV-C envelopes could be selected to allow infection of human cells.

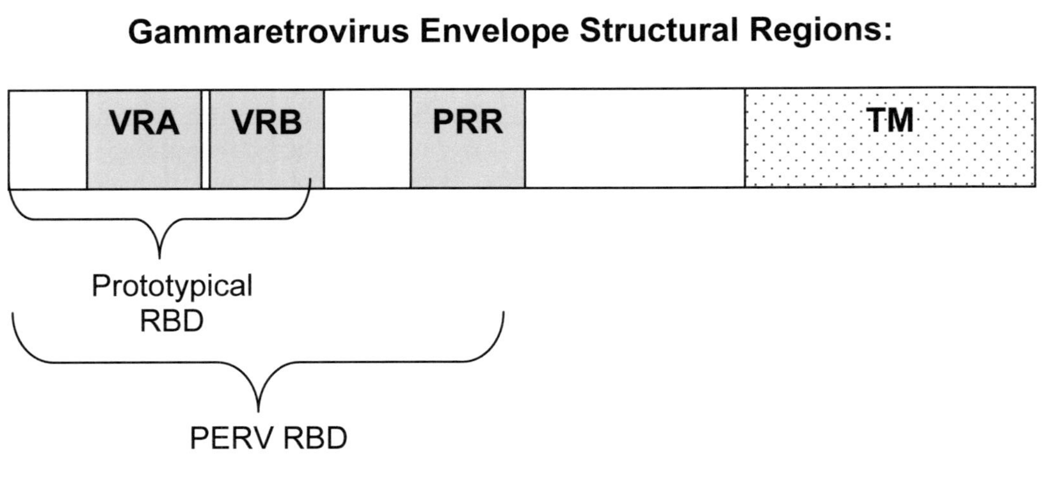

Fig. 2. Receptor Binding Domain for gammaretroviruses and PERV

2.2.4 Human clinical studies

In vitro infection of human cells by PERV, suggesting a risk of cross-species transmission, prompted investigators to perform retrospective studies to determine whether subjects who had previously participated in clinical xenotransplantation trials may have evidence of PERV transmission. Subjects in several different types of xenotransplantation clinical studies were retrospectively analyzed: extracorporeal perfusion through pig cells and organs (Patience, Patton et al. 1998); encapsulated pancreatic islets transplants (Heneine, Tibell et al. 1998; Elliott, Escobar et al. 2007) , and engrafted pig tissues and cells (Paradis, Langford et al. 1999). While one can debate the validity of the various methods chosen (see section 2.1), none of these retrospective studies nor more recent reports of prospectively performed studies (Valdes-Gonzalez, Dorantes et al. 2010) or a survey of abattoir workers (Hermida-Prieto, Domenech et al. 2007) have demonstrated evidence of transmission of PERV to humans exposed to pig xenotransplantation products. Our laboratory also participated in analysis of animal and healthcare workers involved in a clinical xenotransplantation protocol, and did not find any evidence of PERV transmission in that setting (Levy, Argaw et al. 2007). Although the lack of evidence of PERV transmission is encouraging for the safety of these approaches, there are several caveats to interpretation of these negative results: 1) in most recipients, the cells remaining from xenotransplants or extra-corporeally prepared tissues are short lived; 2) assays to monitor PERV transmission may not be sufficiently sensitive and specific; 3) we do not know the best tissue to test for PERV infection, and so for a variety of reasons, investigators sample peripheral blood lymphocytes and serum (Patience, Takeuchi et al. 1997) (FDA 2001). To date, no significant evidence of in vitro infection of human PBMC has been obtained, though that does not rule out the ability of PERV to infect these cells in vivo or their precursor cells in the bone marrow. For a more thorough review of the different clinical studies and methods for assessing human samples for transmission of PERV see (Wilson 2008).

2.2.5 Strategies to prevent or Treat PERV infection in humans

While the actual risk of transmission, replication and pathogenic consequences of exposure to porcine xenotransplantation products to human clinical trial recipients is still not well understood, investigators are pursuing strategies to prevent or treat PERV infection in the xenotransplantation context.

A promising approach that is being investigated is to block expression of PERV RNA using small interfering RNAs (siRNA). Proof of concept studies have been performed in vitro to identify candidate siRNAs; (Karlas, Kurth et al. 2004; Miyagawa, Nakatsu et al. 2005; Dieckhoff, Karlas et al. 2007). Two groups have generated transgenic pigs that express the interfering RNAs (Dieckhoff, Petersen et al. 2008; Ramsoondar, Vaught et al. 2009). Should these prevent PERV expression, use of these as source animals may prevent or reduce transmission of PERV to recipients of porcine xenotransplantation products. While initial reports suggest that the inhibition of gene expression is variable and incomplete, and it is not known whether current levels would prove to be sufficient to prevent PERV transmission, it provides a promising avenue of further effort.

An interesting alternative approach is being evaluated by Yamamoto, et al, using either expression of different mannosidase enzymes or siRNA designed to inhibit expression of the gene encoding the porcine dolichyl-phosphate mannosyl-transferase. They have shown that by essentially altering the mannose residues on the N-linked glycan moieties of PERV envelope, they demonstrate a decrease in PERV infectivity titers on human cells in vitro (Miyagawa, Nakatsu et al. 2006) (Yamamoto, Nakatsu et al. 2010).

In addition to prevention strategies, treatment options are under development. Strategies that are based on using approved anti-HIV drugs have been previously reviewed (Wilson 2008). More recent developments in this field include new monoclonal antibodies with neutralizing activity. Nakaya, et al, have described a monoclonal antibody that potently neutralizes PERV-B, but not PERV-A (Nakaya, Hoshino et al. 2011). Interestingly, the epitope for this neutralizing antibody maps to the proline-rich region, a finding that corresponds to previously described observations that correlate human cell infection with determinants within the PRR (see section 2.2.3). Another group has described two additional neutralizing monoclonal antibodies, one which has been mapped to the C-terminal region of the SU and the other to the TM domain (Chiang, Pan et al. 2007). Unfortunately, the studies are not sufficiently well-described to determine whether either or both of these antibodies recognize and neutralize only PERV-A or if they neutralize both PERV-A and PERV-B, and no follow-up papers have been published on these antibodies since 2007.

3. Conclusion

As highlighted by a recently reported inventory of ongoing human clinical trials in xenotransplantation, there continues to be interest in the clinical application of non-human cells, tissues, and ultimately organs to treat human disease (Sgroi, Buhler et al. 2010). Fortunately, to date, there is no evidence of PERV transmission to any monitored human recipient of a porcine xenotransplantation product. While these data are encouraging, the risks are still unknown should clinical xenotransplantation become successful in reaching the goal of long-term survival of living pig cells, tissues, or organs, in the recipient. The irony of clinical success is that the likelihood of PERV transmission may increase. Therefore, continued investigation into PERV biology and the determinants of human cell infection should be pursued in order to identify avenues to prevent, reduce or treat PERV infection. Until a permissive animal model is developed, gaps in our understanding of the factors affecting in vivo transmission, replication, and potential for pathogenicity cannot be filled. Improved means to detect evidence of PERV infection are also needed.

4. Acknowledgments

The authors wish to thank the many scientific colleagues that have contributed to the work reviewed in this article, and in particular, those additional members of the Wilson laboratory who have provided major contributions to the studies described herein: Winston Colon-Moran, Mariel Figueroa, Malou Gemeniano, Armin Ritzhaupt, Onesmo Mpanju; and our long-time collaborators, Dan Salomon and his colleagues, and Maribeth Eiden, and her colleagues. In addition, we thank Drs. Andrew Byrnes and Keith Wonnacott for their critical reading of the manuscript.

5. References

Akiyoshi, D. E., M. Denaro, et al. (1998). Identification of a full-length cDNA for an endogenous retrovirus of miniature swine. *Journal of Virology* 72(5): 4503-4507, ISSN 022-538X.

Andriamampandry, C., O. Taleb, et al. (2007). Cloning and functional characterization of a gamma-hydroxybutyrate receptor identified in the human brain. *Faseb J* 21(3): 885-95, ISSN 0892-6638.

Archibald, A. L., L. Bolund, et al. (2010). "Pig genome sequence--analysis and publication strategy." *BMC Genomics* 11: 438, ISSN 1471-2164.

Argaw, T., W. Colon-Moran, et al. (2004). Limited infection without evidence of replication by porcine endogenous retrovirus in guinea pigs. *J Gen Virol* 85(Pt 1): 15-9, ISSN 0022-1317.

Argaw, T., M. Figueroa, et al. (2008). "Identification of residues outside of the receptor binding domain that influence the infectivity and tropism of porcine endogenous retrovirus." *J Virol* 82(15): 7483-91, ISSN 022-538X

Argaw, T., A. Ritzhaupt, et al. (2002). Development of a real time quantitative PCR assay for detection of porcine endogenous retrovirus. *J Virol Methods* 106(1): 97-106, ISSN 0166--934.

Armstrong, J. A., J. S. Porterfield, et al. (1971). C-type virus particles in pig kidney cell lines. *Journal of General Virology* 10: 195-198, ISSN 022-1317.

Bellier, B., C. Dalba, et al. (2006). DNA vaccines encoding retrovirus-based virus-like particles induce efficient immune responses without adjuvant. *Vaccine* 24(14): 2643-55, ISSN 0264-410X.

Blusch, J. H., C. Roos, et al. (2000). A polymerase chain reaction-based protocol for the detection of transmission of pig endogenous retroviruses in pig to human xenotransplantation. *Transplantation* 69(10): 2167-72, ISSN 0041-1337.

Bosch, S., C. Arnauld, et al. (2000). Study of full-length porcine endogenous retrovirus genomes with envelope gene polymorphism in a specific-pathogen-free large white swine herd. *Journal of Virology* 74(18): 8575-8581, ISSN 022-538X.

Chiang, C. Y., J. T. Chang, et al. (2005). Characterization of a monoclonal antibody specific to the Gag protein of porcine endogenous retrovirus and its application in detecting the virus infection. *Virus Res* 108(1-2): 139-48, ISSN 0168-1722.

Chiang, C. Y., Y. R. Pan, et al. (2007). Functional epitopes on porcine endogenous retrovirus envelope protein interacting with neutralizing antibody combining sites. *Virology* 361(2): 364-71, ISSN 0042-6822.

Clemenceau, B., S. Lalain, et al. (1999). Porcine endogenous retroviral mRNAs in pancreas and a panel of tissues from specific pathogen-free pigs. *Diabetes and Metabolism (Paris)* 25: 518-525,ISSN 1262-3636.

Deng, Y.-M., B. E. Tuch, et al. (2000). Transmission of porcine endogenous retroviruses in severe combined immunodeficient mice xenotransplanted with fetal porcine pancreatic cells. *Transplantation* 70(7): 1010-1016, ISSN 0041-1337.

Denner, J., H. J. Schuurman, et al. (2009). The International Xenotransplantation Association consensus statement on conditions for undertaking clinical trials of porcine islet products in type 1 diabetes--chapter 5: Strategies to prevent transmission of porcine endogenous retroviruses. *Xenotransplantation* 16(4): 239-48, ISSN 1399-3088.

Denner, J., V. Specke, et al. (2008). No transmission of porcine endogenous retroviruses (PERVs) in a long-term pig to rat xenotransplantation model and no infection of immunosuppressed rats. *Ann Transplant* 13(1): 20-31, ISSN 1425-9524.

Dieckhoff, B., A. Karlas, et al. (2007). Inhibition of porcine endogenous retroviruses (PERVs) in primary porcine cells by RNA interference using lentiviral vectors. *Arch Virol* 152(3): 629-34, ISSN 0304-8608.

Dieckhoff, B., B. Petersen, et al. (2008). Knockdown of porcine endogenous retrovirus (PERV) expression by PERV-specific shRNA in transgenic pigs. *Xenotransplantation* 15(1): 36-45, ISSN 1399-3088.

Dorrschuck, E., N. Fischer, et al. (2011). Restriction of porcine endogenous retrovirus by porcine APOBEC3 cytidine deaminases. *J Virol* 85(8): 3842-57, ISSN 022-538X.

Edamura, K., K. Nasu, et al. (2004). Prevalence of porcine endogenous retrovirus in domestic pigs in Japan and its potential infection in dogs xenotransplanted with porcine pancreatic islet cells. *J Vet Med Sci* 66(2): 129-35, ISSN 0916-7250.

Elliott, R. B., L. Escobar, et al. (2007). Live encapsulated porcine islets from a type 1 diabetic patient 9.5 yr after xenotransplantation. *Xenotransplantation* 14(2): 157-61, ISSN 1399-3088.

Ericsson, T., B. Oldmixon, et al. (2001). Identification of novel porcine endogenous betaretrovirus sequences in miniature swine. *Journal of Virology* 75(6): 2765-2770, ISSN 022-538X.

Ericsson, T. A., Y. Takeuchi, et al. (2003). Identification of receptors for pig endogenous retrovirus. *Proc Natl Acad Sci U S A* 100(11): 6759-64, ISSN 1091-6490.

FDA (2001). Draft Guidance for Industry: Source Animal, Product, Preclinical and Clinical Issues Concerning the Use of Xenotransplantation Products in Humans.

Fiebig, U., O. Stephan, et al. (2003). Neutralizing antibodies against conserved domains of p15E of porcine endogenous retroviruses: basis for a vaccine for xenotransplantation? *Virology* 307(2): 406-13, ISSN 0042-6822.

Fischer, N., U. Krach, et al. (2003). Detection of porcine endogenous retrovirus (PERV) using highly specific antisera against Gag and Env. *Virology* 311(1): 222-8, ISSN 0042-6822.

Galbraith, D. N., H. T. Kelly, et al. (2000). Design and validation of immunological tests for the detection of porcine endogenous retrovirus in biological materials. *J Virol Methods* 90: 115-124, ISSN 0166-0934.

Garkavenko, O., S. Wynyard, et al. (2008). Porcine endogenous retrovirus transmission characteristics from a designated pathogen-free herd. *Transplant Proc* 40(2): 590-3, ISSN 0041-1345.

Gemeniano, M., O. Mpanju, et al. (2006). The infectivity and host range of the ecotropic porcine endogenous retrovirus, PERV-C, is modulated by residues in the C-terminal region of its surface envelope protein. *Virology* 346(1): 108-17. ISSN 0042-6822.

Goila-Gaur, R. and K. Strebel (2008). HIV-1 Vif, APOBEC, and intrinsic immunity. *Retrovirology* 5: 51, ISSN 1742-4690.

Harrison, I., Y. Takeuchi, et al. (2004). Determinants of high titer in recombinant porcine endogenous retroviruses. *J Virol* 78(24): 13871-9, ISSN 022-538X.

Hein, S., V. Prassolov, et al. (2003). Sodium-dependent myo-inositol transporter 1 is a cellular receptor for Mus cervicolor M813 murine leukemia virus. *J Virol* 77(10): 5926-32, ISSN 022-538X.

Heneine, W., A. Tibell, et al. (1998). No evidence of infection with porcine endogenous retrovirus in recipients of porcine islet-cell xenografts. *The Lancet* 352: 695-699, ISSN 0140-6736.

Hermida-Prieto, M., N. Domenech, et al. (2007). Lack of cross-species transmission of porcine endogenous retrovirus (PERV) to transplant recipients and abattoir workers in contact with pigs. *Transplantation* 84(4): 548-50, ISSN 0041-1337.

Herring, C., G. Quinn, et al. (2001). Mapping full-length porcine endogenous retroviruses in a Large White pig. *Journal of Virology* 75(24): 12252-12265, ISSN 022-538X.

Irving, J. M., L. W. S. Chang, et al. (1993). A reverse transcriptase-polymerase chain reaction assay for the detection and quantitation of murine retroviruses. *BioTechnology* 11: 1042-1046, ISSN 1860-7314.

Jaenisch, R. (1982). "Retroviruses and embryogenesis. *Hoppe-Seyler's Zeitschrift fur Physiologische Chemie* 363(11): 1267-1271.

Karlas, A., R. Kurth, et al. (2004). Inhibition of porcine endogenous retroviruses by RNA interference: increasing the safety of xenotransplantation. *Virology* 325(1): 18-23, ISSN 0042-6822.

Krach, U., N. Fischer, et al. (2000). Generation and testing of a highly specific anti-serum directed against porcine endogenous retrovirus nucleocapsid. *Xenotransplantation* 7: 221-229, ISSN 1399-3088.

Laan, L. J. W. v. d., C. Lockey, et al. (2000). Infection by porcine endogenous retrovirus after islet xenotransplantation in SCID mice. *Nature* 407: 90-94, ISSN 0028-0836.

Langford, G., D. Galbraith, et al. (2001). In vivo analysis of porcine endogenous retrovirus expression in transgenic pigs. *Transplantation* 72: 1996, ISSN 0041-1337.

Le Tissier, P., J. P. Stoye, et al. (1997). Two sets of human-tropic pig retroviruses. *Nature* 389: 681-682, ISSN 0028-0836.

Lee, J.-H., G. C. Webb, et al. (2002). Characterizing and mapping porcine endogenous retroviruses in Westran pigs. *Journal of Virology* 76(11): 5548-5556, ISSN 022-538X.

Levy, M. F., T. Argaw, et al. (2007). No evidence of PERV infection in healthcare workers exposed to transgenic porcine liver extracorporeal support. *Xenotransplantation* 14(4): 309-15 ISSN 1399-3088.

Li, Z., Y. Ping, et al. (2004). "Phylogenetic relationship of porcine endogenous retrovirus (PERV) in Chinese pigs with some type C retroviruses. *Virus Res* 105(2): 167-73, ISSN 0168-1702.

Marcucci, K. T., T. Argaw, et al. (2009). Identification of two distinct structural regions in a human porcine endogenous retrovirus receptor, HuPAR2, contributing to function for viral entry. *Retrovirology* 6(1): 3, ISSN 1742-4690.

Martin, U., V. Kiessig, et al. (1998). Expression of pig endogenous retrovirus by primary porcine endothelial cells and infection of human cells. *The Lancet* 352: 692-694, ISSN 0140-6736.

Martina, Y., S. Kurian, et al. (2005). Pseudotyping of porcine endogenous retrovirus by xenotropic murine leukemia virus in a pig islet xenotransplantation model. *Am J Transplant* 5(8): 1837-47, ISSN 1600-6143.

Martina, Y., K. T. Marcucci, et al. (2006). Mice transgenic for a human porcine endogenous retrovirus receptor are susceptible to productive viral infection. *J Virol* 80(7): 3135-46, ISSN 022-538X.

Matthews, A. L., J. Brown, et al. (1999). Development and validation of a western immunoblot assay for detection of antibodies to porcine endogenous retrovirus. *Transplantation* 67(7): 939-943, ISSN 0041-1337

Mattiuzzo, G., M. Matouskova, et al. (2007). Differential resistance to cell entry by porcine endogenous retrovirus subgroup A in rodent species. *Retrovirology* 4: 93, ISSN 1742-4690.

Mattiuzzo, G. and Y. Takeuchi (2010). Suboptimal porcine endogenous retrovirus infection in non-human primate cells: implication for preclinical xenotransplantation. *PLoS One* 5(10): e13203, ISSN 1932-6203.

McIntyre, M. C., B. Kannan, et al. (2003). Detection of porcine endogenous retrovirus in cultures of freshly isolated porcine bone marrow cells. *Xenotransplantation* 10(4): 337-42, ISSN 1399-3088.

Miyagawa, S., S. Nakatsu, et al. (2006). A novel strategy for preventing PERV transmission to human cells by remodeling the viral envelope glycoprotein. *Xenotransplantation* 13(3): 258-63, ISSN 1399-3088.

Miyagawa, S., S. Nakatsu, et al. (2005). "Prevention of PERV infections in pig to human xenotransplantation by the RNA interference silences gene. *J Biochem* 137(4): 503-8, ISSN 0021-924X.

Moalic, Y., Y. Blanchard, et al. (2006). Porcine endogenous retrovirus integration sites in the human genome: features in common with those of murine leukemia virus. *J Virol* 80(22): 10980-8, ISSN 0022-538X.

Moon, H. J., H. K. Kim, et al. (2009). Comparison of the age-related porcine endogenous retrovirus (PERV)expression using duplex RT-PCR. *J Vet Sci* 10(4): 317-22, ISSN 1229-845X.

Morens, D. M. (1994). Antibody-dependent enhancement of infection and the pathogenesis of viral disease. *Clin Infect Dis* 19(3): 500-12, ISSN 1058-4838.

Moscoso, I., M. Hermida-Prieto, et al. (2005). Lack of cross-species transmission of porcine endogenous retrovirus in pig-to-baboon xenotransplantation with sustained depletion of anti-alphagal antibodies. *Transplantation* 79(7): 777-82, ISSN 0041-1337.

Nakaya, Y., S. Hoshino, et al. (2011) Mapping of a neutralizing epitope in the surface envelope protein of porcine endogenous retrovirus subgroup B. *J Gen Virol* 92(Pt 4): 940-4, ISSN 0022-1317.

Neil, S. and P. Bieniasz (2009). Human immunodeficiency virus, restriction factors, and interferon. J *Interferon Cytokine Res* 29(9): 569-80, ISSN 1079-9907.

Niebert, M. and R. R. Tonjes (2003). Analyses of prevalence and polymorphisms of six replication-competent and chromosomally assigned porcine endogenous retroviruses in individual pigs and pig subspecies. *Virology* 313(2): 427-34, ISSN 0042-6822.

Niebert, M. and R. R. Tonjes (2005). Evolutionary spread and recombination of porcine endogenous retroviruses in the suiformes. *J Virol* 79(1): 649-54, ISSN 022-538X.

Oldmixon, B. A., J. C. Wood, et al. (2002). Porcine endogenous retrovirus transmission characteristics of an inbred herd of miniature swine. *Journal of Virology* 76(6): 3045, ISSN 022-538X.

Olsen, C. W. (1993). "A review of feline infectious peritonitis virus: molecular biology, immunopathogenesis, clinical aspects, and vaccination. *Vet Microbiol* 36(1-2): 1-37, ISSN 0378-1135.

Paradis, K., G. Langford, et al. (1999). Search for cross-species transmission of porcine endogenous retrovirus in patients treated with living pig tissue. *Science* 285: 1236-1241, ISSN 0036-8075.

Park, S. J., J. W. Huh, et al. (2010). Analysis of the molecular and regulatory properties of active porcine endogenous retrovirus gamma-1 long terminal repeats in kidney tissues of the NIH-Miniature pig *Mol Cells* 30(4): 319-25, ISSN 1016-8478.

Patience, C., G. S. Patton, et al. (1998). No evidence of pig DNA or retroviral infection in patients with short-term extracorporeal connection to pig kidneys. *The Lancet* 352: 699-701, ISSN 0140-6736.

Patience, C., W. M. Switzer, et al. (2001). Multiple groups of novel retroviral genomes in pigs and related species. *J Virol* 75(6): 2771-5, ISSN 022-538X.

Patience, C., Y. Takeuchi, et al. (1997). Infection of human cells by an endogenous retrovirus of pigs. *Nature Medicine* 3(3): 282-286, ISSN 1078-8956.

PHS (2001). U.S. Public Health Service Guideline on Infectious Disease Issues in Xenotransplantation. *MMWR Morbidity and Mortality Weekly Report Recommendations and Reports* 50: RR-15; www.cdc.gov/mmwr/preview/mmwrhtml/rr5015a1.htm Centers for Disease Control and Prevention 1600 Clifton Rd. Atlanta, GA 30333, USA.

Popp, S. K., D. A. Mann, et al. (2007). Transient transmission of porcine endogenous retrovirus to fetal lambs after pig islet tissue xenotransplantation. *Immunol Cell Biol*, ISSN 0818-9641.

Pyra, H., J. Boni, et al. (1994). Ultrasensitive retrovirus detection by a reverse transcriptase assay based on product enhancement. *Proceedings of the National Academy of Sciences USA* 91: 1544-1548, ISSN 1091-6490.

Ramsoondar, J., T. Vaught, et al. (2009). Production of transgenic pigs that express porcine endogenous retrovirus small interfering RNAs. *Xenotransplantation* 16(3): 164-80, ISSN 1399-3088.

Ritzhaupt, A., L. J. W. v. d. Laan, et al. (2002). Porcine endogenous retrovirus infects but does not replicate in nonhuman primate primary cells and cell lines. *Journal of Virology* 76(22): 11312-11320, ISSN 0022-538X.

Rogel-Gaillard, C., N. Bourgeaux, et al. (1999). Construction of a swine BAC library: application to the characterization and mapping of porcine type C endoviral elements. *Cytogenetics and Cell Genetics* 85: 205-211, ISSN 0301-0171.

Scheef, G., N. Fischer, et al. (2001). The number of a U3 repeat box acting as an enhancer in long terminal repeats of polytropic replication-competent porcine endogenous retroviruses dynamically fluctuates during serial virus passages in human cells. *Journal of Virology* 75(15): 6933-6940, ISSN 022-538X.

Sgroi, A., L. H. Buhler, et al. (2010) International human xenotransplantation inventory. *Transplantation* 90(6): 597-603, ISSN 0041-1337.

Specke, V., R. Plesker, et al. (2009). No in vivo infection of triple immunosuppressed non-human primates after inoculation with high titers of porcine endogenous retroviruses. *Xenotransplantation* 16(1): 34-44, ISSN 1399-3088.

Specke, V., S. J. Tacke, et al. (2001). Porcine endogenous retroviruses: in vitro host range and attempts to establish small animal models. *Journal of General Virology* 82: 837-844, ISSN 022-1317.

Stewart, C., H. Stuhlman, et al. (1982). De novo methylation, expression and infectivity of retroviral genomes introduced into embryonal carcinoma cells. *Proceedings of the National Academy of Sciences USA* 79: 4088-4092, ISSN 1091-6490.

Switzer, W. M., V. Shanmugam, et al. (1999). Polymerase chain reaction assays for the diagnosis of infection with the porcine endogenous retrovirus and the detection of pig cells in human and nonhuman recipients of pig xenografts. *Transplantation* 68(2): 183-188, ISSN 0041-1337.

Takefman, D. M., S. Wong, et al. (2001). Detection and characterization of porcine endogenous retrovirus in porcine plasma and porcine factor VIII. *Journal of Virology* 75(10): 4551-4557, ISSN 022-538X.

Takeuchi, Y., C. Patience, et al. (1998). Host range and interference studies of three classes of pig endogenous retrovirus. *Journal of Virology* 72(12): 9986-9991, ISSN 022-538X.

Valdes-Gonzalez, R., L. M. Dorantes, et al. (2010) No evidence of porcine endogenous retrovirus in patients with type 1 diabetes after long-term porcine islet xenotransplantation. *J Med Virol* 82(2): 331-4, ISSN 0146-6615.

Wilson, C. (2008). Porcine endogenous retroviruses and xenotransplantation. *Cellular and Molecular Life Sciences* 65: 3399-3412, ISSN 1420-682X.

Wilson, C., S. Wong, et al. (1998). Type C retrovirus released from porcine primary peripheral blood mononuclear cells infects human cells. *Journal of Virology* 72(4): 3082-3087, ISSN 022-538X.

Wilson, C. A., S. Laeeq, et al. (2003). Sequence analysis of porcine endogenous retrovirus long terminal repeats and identification of transcriptional regulatory regions. *J Virol* 77(1): 142-9, ISSN 022-538X.

Wilson, C. A., S. Wong, et al. (2000). Extended analysis of the in vitro tropism of porcine endogenous retrovirus. *Journal of Virology* 74(1): 49-56, ISSN 022-538X.

Wood, A., B. L. Webb, et al. (2009). Porcine endogenous retroviruses PERV A and A/C recombinant are insensitive to a range of divergent mammalian TRIM5alpha proteins including human TRIM5alpha. *J Gen Virol* 90(Pt 3): 702-9, ISSN 022-1317.

Wood, J. C., G. Quinn, et al. (2004). Identification of exogenous forms of human-tropic porcine endogenous retrovirus in miniature Swine. *J Virol* 78(5): 2494-501, ISSN 022-538X.

Yamamoto, A., S. Nakatsu, et al. (2010) A newly cloned pig dolichyl-phosphate mannosyl-transferase for preventing the transmission of porcine endogenous retrovirus to human cells. *Transpl Int* 23(4): 424-31, ISSN 0934-0874.

Yang, Y. G., J. C. Wood, et al. (2004). Mouse retrovirus mediates porcine endogenous retrovirus transmission into human cells in long-term human-porcine chimeric mice. *J Clin Invest* 114(5): 695-700, ISSN 0021-9738.

Yin, L., D. Lynch, et al. (1999). Participation of different cell types in the restitutive response of the rat liver to periportal injury induced by allyl alcohol. *J Hepatol* 31(3): 497-507, ISSN 0168-8278.

Yonezawa, A., S. Masuda, et al. (2008). Identification and functional characterization of a novel human and rat riboflavin transporter, RFT1. *Am J Physiol Cell Physiol* 295(3): C632-41,ISSN 0363-6143.